MW00438286

Clinical Aspects and Laboratory

Iron Metabolism, Anemias

Novel concepts
in the anemias of malignancies and renal and rheumatoid diseases

Fifth, enlarged edition

M. Wick
W. Pinggera
P. Lehmann

SpringerWienNewYork

Dr. Manfred Wick

Institute of Clinical Chemistry, Klinikum Grosshadern, University of Munich, Germany

Prim. Univ.-Prof. Dr. Wulf Pinggera

Medical Department, General Hospital, Amstetten, Austria

Dr. Paul Lehmann

Roche Diagnostics GmbH, Mannheim, Germany

© 1991, 1995, 1996, 2000 and 2003 Springer-Verlag/Wien
Printed in Austria

Product Liability: The publisher can give no guarantee for all the information contained in this book. This does also refer to information about drug dosage and application thereof. In every individual case the respective user must check its accuracy by consulting other pharmaceutical literature. The use of registered names, trademarks, etc. in this publication does not imply, even in the absence of a specific statement, that such names are exempt from the relevant protective laws and regulations and therefore free for general use.

Typesetting: GRAPHIK-ART Bauer & Partner, D-67240 Bobenheim-Roxheim
Printing: Adolf Holzhausens Nfg., A-1140 Wien

Printed on acid-free and chlorine free-bleached paper
SPIN: 10918074

With 74 Figures

CIP data applied for

ISBN 3-211-00695-8 Springer-Verlag Wien New York
ISBN 3-211-83357-9 4th ed. Springer-Verlag Wien New York

Foreword

Anemias are a worldwide problem. Severe anemia mainly affects the elderly. The WHO defines anemia as a hemoglobin concentration of less than 12.5 g/dl in women, less than 13.5 g/dl in men, and less than 11.5 g/dl in children (World Health Organization, Nutritional Anemias. Technical Reports Series 1992; 503). According to these criteria, 10 to 20 percent of women and 6 – 30 percent of men above the age of 65 years are anemic. In this book we place new emphasis on the diagnosis and treatment of anemias of chronic disease (ACD) and renal anemias. Nevertheless, iron deficiency remains the most important cause of anemia around the world.

There have been so many advances in the diagnosis and, in particular, the therapy of the anemias in recent years that we felt compelled to extend the spectrum of therapies and diagnostic methods described. Apart from renal and inflammatory anemias, new insights regarding the role of transferrin receptor, the physiology of erythropoietin production and the genetic defect as well as the pathogenesis of hemochromatosis are addressed in this major update of the book.

The authors are grateful to Annett Fahle, Alois Jochum and Dr. Walter Matsui of Roche Diagnostics, Heribert Bauer of Graphik-Art and Michael Katzenberger of Springer-Verlag Wien New York   for their committed cooperation and their expert support in the publication of this book.

M. Wick
W. Pinggera
P. Lehmann

February 2003

Table of Contents

Fundamentals

Fundamentals

Clinical Aspects

Laboratory

Introduction

Disturbances of iron metabolism, particularly iron deficiency and iron redistribution are among the most commonly overlooked or misinterpreted diseases. This is due to the fact that the determination of transport iron in serum or plasma, which used to be the conventional diagnostic test, does not allow a representative estimate of the body's total iron reserves. In the past a proper estimate was only possible by performing costly and invasive determination of storage iron in the bone marrow. However, sensitive, well-standardized immunochemical methods for performing a precise determination of the iron storage protein ferritin in plasma are now available. Since the secretion of this protein correctly reflects the iron stores in the majority of cases, these methods permit fast and reliable diagnoses, particularly of iron deficiency status.

Even non-iron-related causes of anemia can now be identified rapidly using highly sensitive, well standardized methods.

The main physiological relationships are illustrated in Figure 1. The diagnosis of bone marrow diseases should remain the responsibility of experts with experience in hematology. The purpose here is to present the possibilities of non-invasive anemia diagnostics.

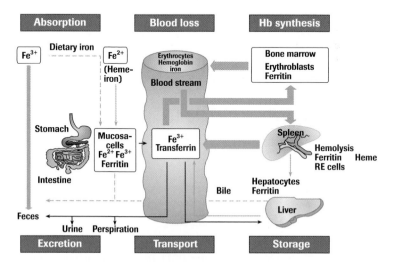

Fig. 1: Physiological principles of iron metabolism

Iron Metabolism

Iron, as a constituent of hemoglobin and cytochromes, is one of the most important biocatalysts in the human body.

Absorption of Iron

The absorption of iron by the human body is limited by the physico-chemical and physiological properties of iron ions, and is possible only when the Fe^{2+}-ion binds with protein (Fig. 2).

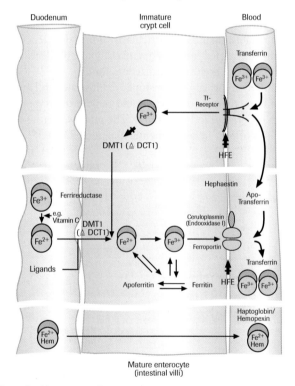

Fig. 2: Intestinal iron resorption

  DMT1: Divalent Metal Transporter; DCT1: Divalent Cation Transporter;
  Tf: Transferrin, HFE: Hemo-Iron; sTfR: Soluble Transferrin Receptor

Iron is absorbed as Fe^{2+} in the duodenum and in the upper jejunum. Since iron in food occurs predominantly in the trivalent form it must first be reduced (apart from the heme-bound Fe^{2+} component), e.g. by ascorbic acid (vitamin C). This explains why only about 10% of the iron in food, corresponding to about 1 mg per day, is generally absorbed. This daily iron intake represents only about 0.25‰ of the body's average total iron pool, which is approximately 4 g; this means that it takes some time to build up adequate reserves of iron. The actual iron uptake fluctuates considerably, depending on absorption-inhibiting and absorption-promoting influences in the upper part of the small intestine. The following factors inhibit absorption in clinically healthy individuals: reduced production of gastric acid, a low level of divalent iron as the result of an unbalanced diet (e.g., in vegetarians), a low level of reducing substances (e.g., ascorbic acid) in the food, or complex formation due to a high consumption of coffee or tea. Conversely, absorption is promoted by a combination of a meat-rich diet with a plentiful supply of heme-bound iron and an acidic, reducing environment due to a high consumption of fruit and vegetables.

The mechanism of iron absorption has become clearer recently. It is assumed to proceed in two stages. When they enter the cells of the mucosa, the Fe^{2+} ions are bound to the transport protein DMT1[*], Nramp2. Before entering the blood plasma they are oxidized to Fe^{3+} by ceruloplasmin (Cp ≙ hephaestin ≙ endoxidase 1 ≙ ferrooxidase), extruded via ferroportin and bound to transferrin [70] (Fig. 2 and Fig. 24).

Within certain limits, the absorption of iron can be adjusted to meet the current iron requirement [144]. Iron deficiency, anemia, and hypoxia lead via increased transferrin and DCT1 synthesis to an increase in the absorption and transport capacity. Conversely, the cells of the mucosa protect the body against alimentary iron overload by storing surplus iron as ferritin. The HFE protein[+], which blocks the transferrin receptor, regulates transferrin-bound iron transport and, therefore, absorption of iron. Immature crypt cells serve as iron sensors, transferrin saturation in the blood controls DMT1 (DCT1) production. Excess iron is excreted after a few days in the course of the physiological cell turnover. The soluble transferrin receptor (sTfR) is an additional regulator of iron uptake derived from erythropoiesis activity.

---

[*] Divalent Ion Metal Transporter (DMT1, formerly referred to as Divalent Cation Transporter, DCT1), and Nramp2, Natural Associated Macrophage Protein 2

[+] Hemo-Iron (HFE) Protein

Fundamentals

Iron Transport

Iron is normally transported via the specific binding of Fe^{3+} by transferrin in blood plasma [42]. The Fe^{3+}-transferrin complex in turn is bound by transferrin receptors to cells of the target organs which allows specific iron uptake according to the individual needs of the various cells. Pronounced non-specific binding to other transport proteins, such as albumin, occurs only in conditions of iron overload with high levels of transferrin saturation.

When there is an excess supply of heme-bound iron, part of the Fe^{2+}-heme complexes may escape oxidation in the cells of the mucosa and be transported to the liver after being bound by haptoglobin or hemopexin.

Transferrin and Iron-Binding Capacity

Transferrin is synthesized in the liver, and has a half-life of 8 to 12 days in the blood. It is a glycoprotein having a molecular weight of 80 kD, and β_1 electrophoretic mobility. Its synthesis in the liver may be increased as a corrective measure, depending on iron requirements and iron reserves. At present little is known about the details of the regulatory mechanisms involved. Transferrin is detectable not only in blood plasma, but also in many interstitial fluids, and a locally synthesized variant with a low neuraminic acid content (β_2 or γ transferrin) is also found in the cerebrospinal fluid. The functional and immunological properties of the many isoforms are substantially the same, the only important difference being the isoelectric point [42]. These forms are therefore of no practical interest with regard either to analytical technique or to the assessment of the iron metabolism (except CDT = carbohydrate deficient transferrin: diagnosis of alcoholism and Beta-2-transferrin: CSF diagnostics). Each transferrin molecule can bind a maximum of 2 F^{3+} ions, corresponding to about 1.5 µg of iron per mg of transferrin.

Transferrin is the most important and specific iron transport protein. Determination of the total specific iron-binding capacity can be measured via the iron and immunological determination of transferrin. In view of its practicability, its low susceptibility to interference, and its high specificity, this method should be used to determine the transferrin-bound iron transport. It has made the determination of the iron saturation = total iron-binding capacity (TIBC) and of the latent iron-binding capacity (LIBC) largely redundant.

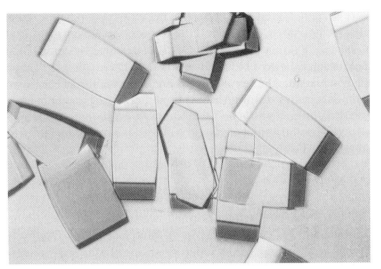

Fig. 3: Transferrin crystals [per Haupt, H. (1990) [72]

Transferrin Saturation (TfS)

Under physiological conditions, transferrin is present in concentrations which exceed the iron-binding capacity normally necessary. About two thirds of the binding sites are therefore unoccupied. The fraction of transferrin binding sites that are not occupied by iron is known as the latent iron-binding capacity (LIBC). It is calculated from the difference between the total iron-binding capacity and the serum iron concentration.

This procedure has been replaced by the determination of the percentage saturation of transferrin (TfS), which does not include non-specific binding of iron by other proteins, so that only the physiologically active iron binding is measured. Fluctuations of the transferrin concentration that are not due to regulatory mechanisms of the iron metabolism can also be eliminated from the assessment in this manner.

Approximately one third of the total iron-binding capacity is normally saturated with iron. Whereas the transferrin concentration remains constant in the range from 2.0 to 4.0 g/l, without any appreciable short-term fluctuations, the transferrin saturation changes quickly with the current iron requirement, and the intake of iron in food. The total quantity of transferrin-bound transport iron in the blood plasma of a healthy adult is only about 4 mg, i.e. only 1% of the body's total iron pool of approximately 4 g.

It is clear from the very low plasma iron concentration and its short-term fluctuations that neither the plasma iron concentration nor the transferrin saturation can provide a true picture of the body's total iron reserves. Assessment of the body's iron reserves is only possible by determination of the storage protein ferritin. The plasma iron concentration and the transferrin saturation only become relevant in the second stage of diagnosis for differentiation of conditions with high plasma ferritin concentrations (see "Disturbances of Iron Distribution and Iron Overload"). The determination of transferrin saturation is preferable to the determination of iron alone, since this eliminates the effects of different blood sampling techniques, different states of hydration in the patient, and different transferrin concentrations. Additionally, the determination of the soluble transferrin receptor (sTfR) has gained importance.

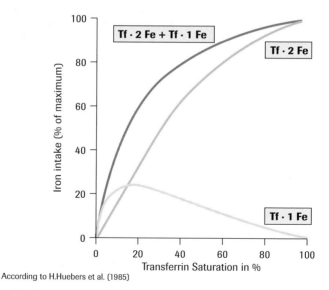

According to H.Huebers et al. (1985)

Fig. 4: Iron intake in the erythroid progenitor cells in dependency on transferrin saturation per Huebers et al. (1990) [87]

Iron Storage

Because of the very limited iron absorption capacity, the average iron requirement can only be met by extremely economical recycling of active iron. Iron is stored in the form of ferritin or its semi-crystalline condensation product hemosiderin in the liver, spleen, and bone marrow. In principle, every cell has the ability to store an excess of iron through ferritin synthesis [145]. The fundamental mechanisms are identical for all types of cells (Fig. 5).

The transferrin-Fe^{3+} complex is bound to the transferrin receptor of the cell membrane. Iron uptake can therefore be regulated by the transferrin receptor expression. Iron directly induces the synthesis of apoferritin, the iron-free protein shell of ferritin, on the cytoplasmic ribosomes. In the majority of metabolic situations, a representative fraction of the ferritin synthesized is released into the blood plasma [37]. The ferritin concentration correctly reflects the amount of storage iron available (*exception:* disturbances of iron distribution). This has been verified experimentally by comparison with iron determinations in bone-marrow aspirates [97]. In clinical diagnosis ferritin should be determined as the parameter of first choice for the assessment of iron reserves, e.g. in the identification of the cause of an anemia.

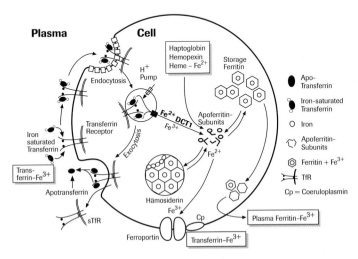

Fig. 5: Cellular iron storage and ferritin synthesis

The relationship between iron reserves and serum ferritin is valid for all stages of iron deficiency, the normal state and almost all forms of iron overload. The rule of thumb is:

---

1 µg/L of serum ferritin corresponds to approximately 10 mg of stored iron

---

This can be used not only to estimate the amount of iron required to replenish stores during iron deficiency but also to estimate iron excess in the case of iron overload as well as for the monitoring of the course of these disorders.

In addition to the general mechanisms of cellular iron storage and uptake, the liver and the spleen also have specialized metabolic pathways. Hepatocytes, for example, can convert haptoglobin-bound or hemopexin-bound hemoglobin-Fe^{2+} from intravascular hemolysis or from increased heme absorption into ferritin-Fe^{3+} storage iron. On the other hand, the regular lysis of senescent erythrocytes and the associated conversion of Fe^{2+}-hemoglobin into Fe^{3+}-ferritin storage iron takes place mainly in the reticuloendothelial cells of the spleen. Ceruloplasmin also plays a decisive role in the oxidation of Fe^{2+} into Fe^{3+}.

Ferritin and Isoferritins

Ferritin is a macromolecule having a molecular weight of at least 440 kD (depending on the iron content), and consists of a protein shell (apoferritin) of 24 subunits and an iron core containing an average of about 2500 Fe^{3+} ions (in liver and spleen ferritin) (Fig. 6). Ferritin tends to form oligomers (approx. 10 to 15%), and when present in excess in the cells of the storage organs it tends to condense, with formation of semicrystalline hemosiderin in the lysosomes.

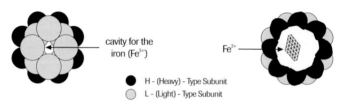

cavity for the iron (Fe^{3+})

Fe^{3+}

● H - (Heavy) - Type Subunit
○ L - (Light) - Type Subunit

Fig. 6: Structure of the ferritin molecule

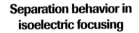

Separation behavior in isoelectric focusing

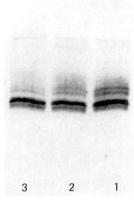

1. Heart Ferritin
2. Liver Ferritin
3. Spleen Ferritin

3   2   1

Fig. 7: Isoelectric focusing of acidic (top) and basic isoferritins (bottom)

At least 20 isoferritins can be distinguished using isoelectric focusing [6] (Fig. 7). The microheterogeneity is due to differences in the contents of acidic H subunits and slightly basic L subunits. The basic isoferritins are responsible for long-term iron storage, and are found mainly in the liver, spleen, and bone marrow. The storage ferritins of this group can be measured by the commercially available immunoassay methods, which are standardized against liver and/or spleen ferritin preparations. Their determination provides a reliable picture of the iron reserves [40]. The 3rd International Standard for recombinant L-Ferritin has been available since 1997 [185].

Acidic isoferritins are found mainly in myocardium, placenta, and tumor tissue, and in smaller quantities also in the depot organs. They have lower iron contents, and presumably function as intermediaries for the transfer of iron in synthetic processes [89]. Unlike the basic isoferritins, they exhibit practically no response to the commercially available immunoassay methods. The use of suitable highly specific antisera would be necessary for their selective determination (Fig. 8).

Table 1: Clinically important characteristics of the depot protein ferritin

Ferritin
Iron storage protein Molecular weight > 440 kD

Isoferritins	
Basic L-isoferritins Rich in iron	Acidic H-isoferritins Poor in iron
Stored in: Liver Spleen Bone marrow	Stored in: Placenta Heart Tumors

Plasma ferritin is basic and correlates with the body's total iron stores (exception: disturbances of iron distribution)

Iron Distribution

It can be seen from Fig. 8 that most (about 2500 mg) of the total iron pool is contained in the erythrocytes as hemoglobin-bound active iron. A further 400 mg is required as active iron in myoglobin and various enzymes. If the supply of iron is adequate (men and postmenopausal women), considerably quantities are also stored as basic ferritin (approx. 800 to 1200 mg) in the depot organs liver, spleen, and bone marrow [6]. Only a small fraction (approx. 4 mg) of the body's total iron pool is in the form of transferrin-bound transport iron in the blood plasma. It is thus once again clear that the measurement of iron in plasma does not provide a true picture of the available storage iron (Fig. 10).

Fundamentals

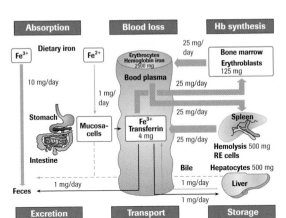

Fig. 8: Balance of iron metabolism

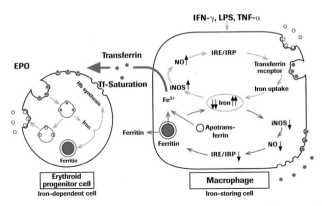

Fig. 9: Normal state. Model of the autoregulatory loop between iron metabolism and the NO/NOS pathway in activated monocytes/macrophages and supply of an iron dependent cell. Weiss, G., et al. (1997) [195].

Abbreviations: IFN-γ, interferon γ, iNOS = inducible nitric oxide synthase; IRE, iron-responsive element; IRP/IRP: high-affinity binding of iron-regulatory protein (IRP) to IREs; LPS, lipopolysaccharide; TNF-α, tumor necrosis factor α; ↑ and ↓ indicate increase or decrease of cellular responses, respectively.

Iron stored as ferritin within an iron-storing cell is released and bound to apotransferrin, followed by its transport to the iron-dependent cell.

The cytoplasmic membrane contains transferrin receptors to which the iron-carrying transferrin binds.

The endosome migrates into the cytoplasm where it releases iron.

The free iron is either used as functional iron or is stored as ferritin.

Explanation of signs: ⌣ transferrin receptor ● iron-carrying transferrin
○ apotransferrin ⊙ ferritin

The autoregulation of iron metabolism and its effect on the NO/NOS pathway in activated monocytes and macrophages is depicted in Fig. 9 [195]. The illustration in Fig. 10 shows the close relationship between cell-cell interactions in the differentiation of T-cells from TH1 and TH2 cells, and macrophage activation of CD4+TH0 cells and TH1 cells [132]. When iron status is normal, TH1 cells are not activated nor are inflammatory reactions triggered in the activated macrophages, because the IL-1, IL-12 cytokines required for T-cell activation are secreted in concentrations that do not trigger an inflammatory response (Fig. 10). See also page 87 ff. Conversely in the absence of inflammation there is no effect on iron distribution in macrophages.

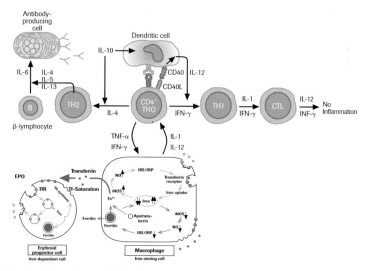

Fig. 10: Normal state. Cell-cell interactions of cytokines in the differentiation of T-cells from TH1 and TH2 cells, and influence by the autoregulation of iron metabolism and the NO/NOS pathway in activated macrophages. Moldawer, et al. (1997) [132] and Weiss, et al. (1997) [195]

Iron Requirement and Iron Balance

The iron distribution described is valid only for healthy adult men and for postmenopausal women, who have an iron replacement requirement of not more than 1 mg per day. The iron requirement is up to 5 mg per day for adolescents, menstruating women and blood donors, as well as in cases of extreme physical stress due to anabolic processes or iron losses. Pregnant women require additional quantities of iron of up to 7 mg per day. This increased requirement cannot always be met by increased absorption, even with an adequate supply of iron in the food. The result is a progressive depletion of the iron stores, which can lead to manifest iron deficiency if the supply of iron remains inadequate over a long period. Where iron requirement is increased for the reasons given above, transferrin receptor expression is up-regulated. At the same time the concentration of the soluble transferrin receptor in the plasma rises accordingly. In most cases, increased erythropoiesis is the main reason for the increased iron requirement.

Unlike the absorption of iron, the excretion of iron is not actively regulated. A total of up to approximately. 1 mg of iron per day is lost under normal conditions. Iron balance is therefore only partially capable of being regulated via iron intake. The internal turnover of iron resulting from the degradation of senescent erythrocytes, at about 20 to 25 mg per day, is much higher than the daily intake and excretion of iron. The individual requirement to newly synthesize hemoglobin and enzymes can therefore only be met by extremely economical recyc-ling of available reserves.

Transferrin Receptor (TfR)

All tissues and cells which require iron regulate their iron uptake by expression of the transferrin receptor on the surface of the cell. Since most of the iron is required for hemoglobin synthesis in the precursor cells of erythropoiesis in the bone marrow, approximately 80% of the transferrin receptors of the body can be found on these cells. All cells are capable of regulating individual transferrin receptor expression according to the current iron requirement or the supply of iron at the cell level. The transferrin receptor is a dimeric protein with a molecular weight of approximately 190 000 daltons. Each of the two sub-units is capable of binding a molecule of transferrin [186]. In iron metabolism the transferrin receptor has a major role in supplying the cell with iron. Fe ion transport in the blood occurs by the specific binding of Fe^{3+} ions to transferrin; a maximum of two Fe^{3+} ions can be transported per protein molecule. The affinity of the membrane-bound transferrin receptor to the transferrin-Fe complex in the weakly alkaline pH of the blood depends on the Fe load of the transferrin. It is low when transferrin saturation is low (< 15%). A maximum is reached when the Tf load is 2 Fe ions (Fig. 11).

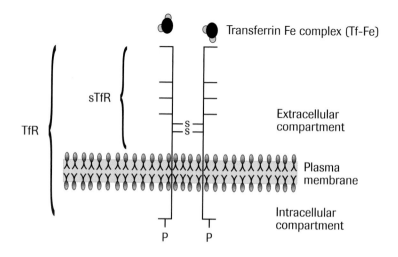

Fig. 11: Scheme of the TfR and sTfR molecule (Punnonen et al., 1997 [147])

A representative proportion of the membrane-bound transferrin receptors is released into the plasma as soluble transferrin receptor (sTfR).

The TfR-Tf-Fe complex is channeled through a pH gradient into the cell by the "endocytic residue". The change from the alkaline pH of the blood into the acidic pH of the endosome changes the binding situation: Iron ions dissociate spontaneously from transferrin while the bond between Tf and TfR remains intact (Fig. 12). Only when the TfR-Tf complex returns to the cell membrane does the pH change into the alkaline pH of the blood cause the complex to dissociate. The transferrin reenters the plasma and is again available for Fe transport [4, 55].

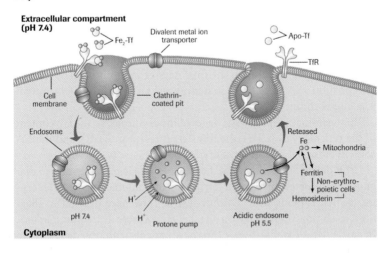

Fig. 12: Iron uptake in the cell aided by the transferrin-transferrin receptor complex by the "endocytic residue". (N.C. Andrews, 1999 [4])

Soluble Transferrin Receptor (sTfR)

Expression of the transferrin receptor (TfR) is regulated by the intracellular concentration of the iron ions. If the iron requirement of the cell is large, but the iron concentration is small, TfR expression and, at the same time, the concentration of the soluble serum transferrin receptor (sTfR) increases. Conversely, where there is iron overload, both the TfR concentration and the concentration of soluble TfR are low. As the concentration of the soluble transferrin receptor reflects the total number of cell-bound transferrin receptors and these, in turn, are mainly to be found on erythropoietic cells in the bone marrow, in a healthy person with an adequate iron supply the transferrin-receptor concentration is one of the best indicators of erythropoietic activity [11, 35]. The sTfR concentration depends on the iron requirement and erythropoietic activity. Increased levels of sTfR are therefore found in patients with iron deficiency and increased erythropoiesis. The cell-bound transferrin receptor on the precursor cells of erythropoiesis is also called the CD71 antigen. A high concentration of cellular RNA remains there after the transferrin receptor has been expressed in high concentrations. These two states are necessary to channel a sufficient quantity of transferrin-bound iron into the erythrocytes and to synthesize the necessary Hb by the RNA residue. About 20 to 30 % of the total cellular erythrocytic Hb is formed in this manner in the final days of maturation. The nucleic acid portion (NA) is neglible in mature erythrocytes while Hb content is at a maximum.

In the immature precursor stages of the erythrocytes, the Hb content of the reticulocytes (CHr), the transferrin receptor (sTfR), and the NA content are equal indicators of erythropoietic activity.

Iron deficiency in otherwise healthy persons is relatively easy to diagnose by the determination of ferritin and the soluble transferrin receptor (sTfR). Patients with "chronic disease" are more difficult to diagnose, as chronic diseases have a direct effect on these iron status markers. In particular, a chronic disease can cause patients with iron deficiency to have normal serum ferritin values, while serum iron values are reduced in patients with sufficient iron reserves. In this group of patients, it has been demonstrated that determination of the soluble transferrin receptor (sTfR) in serum is comparable to determination in bone-marrow aspirate when it comes to identifying patients with iron deficiency [147, 148]. Expression of the transferrin receptor is directly proportional to the iron requirement in the cell, i.e. TfR is elevated in patients with iron deficiency. The level of sTfR in the serum is also elevated, as it is proportional to the total amount of transferrin receptor in the cell [35, 36].

Iron Losses

A total of about 1 mg of iron per day is excreted via the intestine, urine and perspiration. Menstruating women lose 30 to 60 ml of blood, containing about 15 to 30 mg of iron, every month. With an adequate supply of iron in the diet, these losses can be replaced through increased absorption.

Hypermenorrhea, particularly in combination with an unbalanced diet, is a cause of iron deficiency. Another cause is frequent blood donations.

Erythropoiesis

Physiological Cell Maturation

An adult has on average 5 liters of blood and an erythrocyte count of $5 \times 10^6/\mu l$, giving a total erythrocyte count of 2.5×10^{13}. Since the mean life span of an erythrocyte is normally 120 days, about 2×10^{11} new erythrocytes need to be formed daily to maintain this erythrocyte pool. For this to happen, about 20-30% of the medullary stem cells must be differentiated to cells of erythropoiesis. Different stages in maturation can be identified on the basis of cell morphology and biochemical capacity. The immature nucleated cells, such as preerythrobalsts and erythroblasts (macroblasts), with their high DNA, RNA and protein synthesizing capacity, ensure that there is adequate proliferation of erythrocyte precursors under stimulation by erythropoietin.

However, this requires the availability of sufficient cobalamin (vitamin B_{12}) and folic acid, which acts as carriers of C1 units in the synthesis of nucleic acid. Vitamin B_{12} (daily requirement about 3 µg) is derived mainly from foods of animal origin. Absorption in the terminal ileum calls for production of sufficient intrinsic factor by the parietal cells in the fundus/body region of the stomach. By contrast, folic acid (daily requirement > 200 µg) is derived mainly from foods of plant origin and, probably for the most part, via synthesis by intestinal bacteria, and absorbed in the jejunum. Considerable amounts of both vitamins are stored in the liver.

Hemoglobin synthesis then occurs at the normoblast stage of maturation, which is shown morphologically in the conversion of basophilic into oxyphilic normoblasts (with red cytoplasm). Once the normoblast is filled with hemoglobin, the cell nucleus and mitochondria can be expelled, and the cell which leaves the bone marrow is known as a reticulocyte. It thereby loses most of its biochemical synthesis capabilities and its ability to divide, and subsequently circulates in the peripheral blood as a highly specialized, mature erythrocyte serving almost exclusively for the transportation of oxygen. All forms of anemia that are not primarily hemolytic thus have their roots in disturbances of cell proliferation or hemoglobin synthesis or in deficiencies at bone-marrow level. The reticulocyte count thereby serves as the simplest indicator of hemogenesis.

Hemoglobin Synthesis

Hemoglobin consists of over 90% protein; in the fetus this is made up of 2 α- and 2 γ-polypeptide chains (known as HbF), whereas in adults it is predominantly 2 α- and 2 β-chains (HbA0), with a small portion of 2 α- and 2 γ–chains (HbA2).

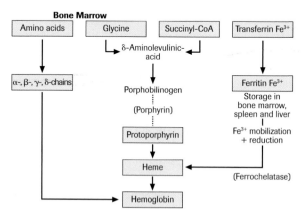

Fig. 13: Hemoglobin synthesis

Each of these chains carries a heme as prosthetic group, which in turn is capable of binding an oxygen molecule. The total molecular weight of this tetramer is about 68,000 daltons.

The formation of the normal quaternary structure is dependent on the regular synthesis not only of the protein chains but also of the porphyrin component, and in particular on the adequate adhesion of the heme and protein components by means of iron which also guarantees oxygen binding [162]. An overview of hemoglobin synthesis is given in Fig. 13.

Erythropoietin

Erythropoietin (EPO) is a glycoprotein with a molecular weight of 34,000 daltons (Fig. 14). As hematopoietic growth factor, the hormone regulates the rate of red cell-production, keeping the circulating red cell mass constant. EPO is produced in response to a hypoxia signal as a result of a decrease in the oxygen tension in the blood [166].

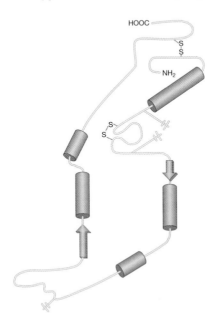

Fig. 14: Molecular biology of erythropoietin (from: Wieczorek K, Hirth P, Schöpe KB, Scigalla P, Krüger D (1989). In: Gurland S (ed), Innovative Aspekte der klinischen Medizin. Springer, Berlin Heidelberg New York Tokyo, pp 55-70)

EPO, which is produced primarily in the kidney, stimulates the proliferation of the bone marrow erythroid progenitor cells, accelerates their differentiation into mature erythrocytes, promotes hemoglobin synthesis and TfR expression [195], shortens the maturation process of erythroblasts, and stimulates the release of reticulocytes from the bone marrow (Fig. 15).

In the kidney, EPO is formed in peritubular interstitial cells in the renal cortex, which act as sensors of the intracapillary oxygen content. These cells proliferate if pO_2 drops slightly as a result of hypoxia or if there is a reduction in renal blood flow. EPO synthesis in each cell increases. An increase in EPO-mRNA precedes increased synthesis.

EPO is bound primarily via receptors to erythroid progenitor cells up to the erythroblast stage. Even BFU-E (burst forming units) have EPO receptors; they increase up to the CFU-E (colony forming unit) stage. Cell maturation stages between CFU-E and proerythroblasts have the highest density of EPO receptors. Extremely few receptors are found on the orthochromatic normoblast.

After uptake, EPO is degraded in the cell. Whether or not the EPO receptors remain intact is unclear. EPO acts on erythroid precursor cells, regardless of their division and differentiation. It delays the degradation of nucleic acids (NA) in CFU-E.

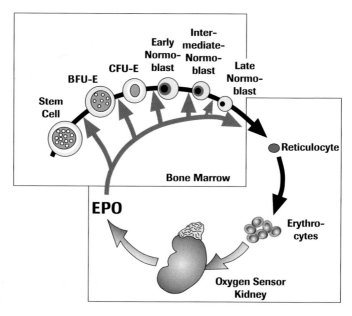

Fig. 15: Stimulation and regulation of erythrocyte formation by erythropoietin

Up to now the determination of erythropoietin has been of limited diagnostic value. It can be used, for example, to differentiate between primary causes of erythrocytosis such as polycythemia vera and secondary causes such as increased production of erythropoietin, e.g. in lung diseases with hypoxia or certain tumors. In renal anemia, decreased erythropoietin production can usually be assumed to be the cause. In every case where a true erythropoietin deficiency does not exist but rather an inadequate erythropoietin response, i.e. anemia with normal erythropoietin levels, the determination of erythropoietin is suitable for detecting this inadequate erythropoietin response.

> **The reference range for EPO in serum is 5 to 25 U/L.**
> **1 mg EPO equals 50 000 IU.**

Increased EPO levels in serum are measured in patients with cardiac and pulmonary insufficiency, for example, and in patients with erythrocytosis with high oxygen affinity (e.g. HbF). EPO levels typically increase in serum when the level of Hb falls below 12 g/dL.

A decrease in EPO levels is observed in patients with impaired renal function. Patients with chronic renal insufficiency develop anemia and erythropoiesis is inadequate. Additional extracorporal factors (e.g. hemolysis) can also play a role in the development of anemia.

Phagocytosis of Old Erythrocytes

During the physiological aging process the circulating erythrocytes lose more and more of their terminal neuraminic acid residues of their membrane glycoproteins, which leads to increased binding of IgG. This changed membrane surface structure is now the signal to the macrophages of above all the spleen and the liver to start phagocytosis of the old erythrocytes. This occurs physiologically after about 120 days, so that 0.8% of the erythrocyte pool or 1×10^{11} erythrocytes are lysed each day, maintaining equilibrium with the daily new formation rate.

Hemoglobin Degradation

The globin content of the hemoglobin is hydrolyzed by proteases to amino acids which are either available for the synthesis of new proteins or are further degraded by deamination. The iron which is released must be reused extremely economically and, so as to avoid toxic effects, oxidized and incorporated into basic isoferritins for interim storage. In this process, the macrophages of the RES (reticuloendothelial system) in particular in the spleen serve as short-term stores from which ferritin-bound iron can be remobilized and transported via transferrin to the bone marrow for the synthesis of new hemoglobin. At a physiological hemolysis rate, about 6.5 g per day of hemoglobin is catabolized, and the corresponding quantity newly synthesized, giving an iron turnover of about 25 mg/24 h [156, 162]. Given a daily iron absorption of 1 mg, this again shows clearly that the iron requirement can be met only after careful utilization.

The porphyrin ring of the heme is degraded to bilirubin via biliverdin. Since nonglucuronidized bilirubin is not water-soluble, it must first be transported in albumin-bound form to the liver where it is conjugated with glucuronic acid and thus converted into a form which can be eliminated with the bile (Fig. 16). ´

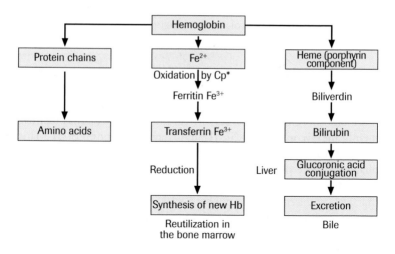

Fig. 16: Hemoglobin degradation (*Cp = ceruloplasmin)

Disturbances of Iron Metabolism/ Disturbances of Erythropoiesis and Hemolysis

Disturbances of the Body's Iron Balance

An impaired iron balance of the body can frequently be described as a discordant regulation of synthesis of ferritin, the iron storage protein, on the one hand, and of the transferrin receptor, the indicator of iron demand and erythropoietic activity, on the other. This is particularly true if iron deficiency or iron overload are not complicated by additional diseases such as inflammations, tumors or renal failure.

In true storage iron deficiency a lack of intracellular iron ions leads to downregulation of apoferritin synthesis and consequently also to a decreased release of ferritin into the peripheral blood. To compensate for this, expression of transferrin receptor is upregulated in order to meet the iron demand of the cell despite depleted iron reserves and low transferrin saturation. This leads to an increased concentration of soluble transferrin receptor (sTfR) in blood. This discordant regulation may be found already in latent iron deficiency, preceding the development of a hypochromic anemia. If these changes are not yet very marked, in doubtful cases the ratio of transferrin receptor and ferritin concentrations may show this state more clearly. The transport iron, determined by measuring the transferrin saturation, additionally contributes to the staging.

Opposite dysregulations are found in simple iron overload (for instance hereditary hemochromatosis) unless associated with chronic inflammations, malignant disease, ineffective erythropoiesis or hemolysis.

The discordant regulation of ferritin and transferrin receptor production is impaired, however, in cases of iron redistribution in chronic inflammations or tumors, in cases of increased erythropoietic activity due to hemolysis or erythropoietin therapy or in bone marrow diseases with increased but ineffective erythropoiesis (for instance myelodysplastic syndrome). This unusual reaction pattern can, however, be used to diagnose an increased iron demand despite sufficient or even increased iron reserves, particularly under erythropoietin therapy.

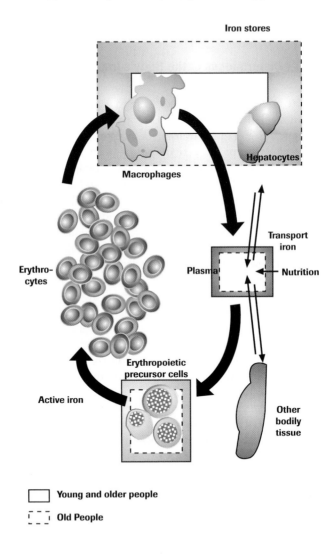

Fig. 17: Functional iron, transport iron, iron stores in iron metabolism

Table 2: Indicators of disturbances of iron balance - ferritin versus soluble transferrin receptor (sTfR)

	Ferritin	Transferrin-saturation	sTfR	Reticulo-cytes	MCV	Hemo-globin

Iron deficiency
   latent
   manifest
	↓
	↓ ↓
		↓
		↓ ↓
			↑
			↑ ↑
				n - ↓
				↓
					n - ↓
					↓
						n
						↓

Iron redistribution (ACD)	n - ↑ ↑	↓	n - ↑	↓	n - ↓	↓
Renal anemia (without EPO)	n - ↑	↓	n - ↓	↓	n	↓
Iron utilization-defects (incl. MDS)	n - ↑	n - ↑	n - ↑	↓	↓ - ↑	↓
Hemolysis	n - ↑	n - ↑	↑	↑	n - ↑	n - ↓
Iron overload (hereditary, e.g. hemochromatosis)	↑ - ↑ ↑	↑ - ↑ ↑	↓	n	n	n

MDS = myelodysplastic syndrome
ACD = anemia of chronic disease

Iron Deficiency

Even under physiological conditions, an increased iron requirement and/or increased loss of iron (in puberty, in menstruating or pregnant women, in blood donors or in competitive athletes) can lead to iron deficiency. With an unbalanced diet, the iron balance is often upset by a shortage of absorbable iron.

The first stage is a shortage of depot iron (prelatent iron deficiency), which is reflected in a reduced plasma ferritin concentration. When the iron stores are completely empty, a transport iron deficiency develops, though hemoglobin synthesis is still adequate at this stage (latent iron deficiency). With additional stress or loss of iron, however, this condition may progress into a manifest iron deficiency with hypochromic microcytic anemia. The latter is more often associated with a pathological chronic loss of blood, especially as a result of ulcers or tumors of the gastrointestinal and urogenital tracts, or with disturbances of iron absorption (e.g., after resections in the upper gastrointestinal tract or chronic inflammatory diseases of the small intestine).

All forms of iron deficiency can be identified by the following pattern of laboratory findings: reduced ferritin concentration with a compensating increase in the transferrin concentration, low transferrin saturation, and increased concentration of soluble transferrin receptor (sTfR) in different levels of intensity. The reduced ferritin concentration is the only reliable indicator of iron-deficient conditions. It enables the latter to be distinguished from other causes of hypochromic anemia, such as chronic inflammations and tumors [77] (Table 2).

Iron deficiency, of whatever cause, also leads to increased transferrin receptor expression and accordingly to an increased concentration of the soluble transferrin receptor (sTfR) in the plasma. In these cases there is no longer any correlation between transferrin receptor and erythropoietic activity. All forms of simple depot iron deficiency can be detected with an adequate degree of certainty by a decreased plasma ferritin concentration. In iron deficiency due to bleeding, inflammations or tumors this may be masked. On the other hand, in cases with sufficient iron reserves and only so-called functional iron deficiency, i.e. disturbances of iron utilization, an increasing concentration of soluble transferrin receptors may give an early indication of the relative shortage of iron of erythropoiesis or deficient iron mobilization. In these cases of complicated storage or functional iron deficiency, sTfR may show the increased iron demand.

A correct diagnosis of iron deficiency is critical for the successful treatment of anemias. Experience shows that often the only possibility is to classify the diagnosis as either certain iron deficiency, absence of iron deficiency, or possible iron deficiency. Patients classified in the latter category primarily have anemias that occur in conjunction with infections, acute chronic inflammation or malignant tumors. A majority of these patients have an acute phase reaction with an increase in C-reactive protein (CRP) to above 5 mg/l.

The objective of laboratory testing is to:
- Detect the subclinical iron deficiency and administer early therapy to prevent systemic complications of this disease;
- Identify anemias that are based on uncomplicated iron deficiency (increased menstruation, chronic intestinal bleeding, nutritive iron deficiency), because they respond very quickly to iron therapy;

• Detect inadequate iron supply of erythropoiesis in anemias where disturbance of iron distribution is paramount (anemias in infections and inflammations, and tumor anemia).

Disturbances of Iron Distribution

Malignant neoplasias and chronic inflammations lead to a shortage of transport- and active iron, with simultaneous relative overloading of the iron stores [31]. When tumors are present, the disturbance of the iron distribution is further influenced by the increased iron requirement of the tumor tissue. These conditions, like manifest iron deficiency, are characterized by microcytic anemia, elevated ferritin and low transferrin saturation values. Genuine iron deficiency is distinguished by reduced ferritin and elevated transferrin receptor concentrations, and reduced transferrin saturation.

The elevated ferritin concentration in these cases is not representative of the body's total iron reserves, but indicates the redistribution to the iron-storing tissue. The low transferrin saturation distinguishes disturbances of iron distribution from genuine iron overload conditions.

In the presence of tumors, the disturbed iron distribution with increased release of iron-rich basic isoferritins into the blood plasma is accompanied by separate synthesis of mainly acidic iron-poor isoferritins. Only a small fraction of the acidic isoferritins is normally detected by commercially available immunoassay methods, but at very high concentrations they can lead to raised ferritin concentrations. The total ferritin concentration is therefore underestimated in the presence of tumors.

A non-representative elevation of the plasma ferritin concentration is also found in patients with cell necrosis of the iron-storage organs, e.g. in liver diseases. Transferrin saturation is also elevated in this case, however.

In most of the iron distribution disturbances, there is a relative shortage in the amount of iron supplied to the erythropoietic cells, together with reduced erythropoietic activity. Correspondingly, transferrin receptor expression is usually normal. In the case of rapidly growing tumors, it can also be elevated as a result of the increased iron requirement of the tumor cells.

A very rare hereditary form of iron redistribution is caused by atransferrinemia. The lack of transferrin-bound iron transport leads to low iron concentrations in plasma and a reduced supply of all iron consuming organs. The transport function is taken over nonspecifically by other proteins such as albumin, leading to an uncontrolled deposition of iron in cells, which is not regulated according to demand by transferrin receptor expression.

Anemias of Malignancies and Anemias of Chronic Diseases (ACD) in Inflammations

As described above, iron redistribution with a relative over-loading of iron stores and concomitant relative iron deficiency of erythropoietic cells (as a consequence of reduced transferrin synthesis) can occur mainly in tumor anemias and chronic inflammation (infections and primarily rheumatic diseases). Transferrin is an anti-acute-phase protein, of course, the synthesis of which is down-regulated in the presence of said diseases as a result of an evolutionary natural selection process. Susceptibility to bacterial infections decreases in the presence of reduced availability of transport iron, because bacteria and other causative agents of infection also require large quantities of iron to replicate. The reduced availability of iron therefore acts as a protective mechanism on the one hand and, on the other, it represents a major pathomechanism of the development of anemias of infection. If the redistribution of iron is predominant, then hypochromic anemia is highly probable and can be differentiated from iron deficiency anemia by ferritin and soluble transferrin receptor (sTfR) assays.

Apart from down-regulation of transferrin, a second cause of iron redistribution in inflammations has recently been identified [31, 32, 91, 92, 196]. Increased production of cytokines such as IFN-γ and TNF-α, mediated by nitric oxide (NO), stimulates iron uptake in macrophages by increased transferrin receptor expression. As a consequence, increased iron uptake induces increased intracellular ferritin synthesis, which in turn causes enhanced ferritin release into plasma. Increased iron storage in macrophages in ACD and tumors draws iron from transferrin, which is already reduced. In contrast to true iron overload, this kind of iron redistribution is characterized by a low transferrin saturation. This second mechanism increases the iron deficiency in all iron-consuming cells in the body (Fig. 18).

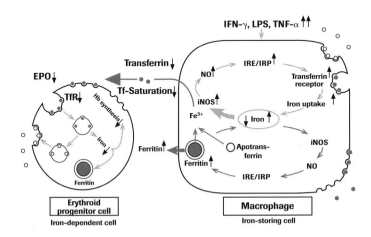

Fig. 18: Iron redistribution in ACD

Model of the autoregulatory loop between iron metabolism and the NO/NOS pathway in activated monocytes/macrophages and supply of an iron-dependent cell.

Weiss, G. et al. (1997) [196]

Abbreviations: IFN-γ, interferon γ; iNOS = inducible nitric oxide synthase; IRE, iron-responsive element; IRE/IRP high-affinity binding of iron-regulatory protein (IRP) to IREs; LPS, lipopolysaccharide; TNF-α, tumor necrosis factor α; $\uparrow$ and $\downarrow$ indicate increase or decrease of cellular responses, respectively.

Supply of an iron-dependent cell.

Iron stored as ferritin within an iron-storing cell is released to transferrin, and then carried to the iron-requiring cell.
The cytoplasmic membrane of tissue cells contains transferrin receptors to which the iron-carrying transferrin binds.

The endosome migrates into the cytoplasm where it releases iron.

The endosome returns to the cytoplasmic membrane and apotransferrin is released into the extracellular space.

Explanation of signs: $\cup$ transferrin receptor ● iron-carrying transferrin
                       ○ apotransferrin ⊙ ferritin

The availability of iron is reduced in particular for the synthesis of hemoglobin. This vicious circle can possibly be broken by substitution of erythropoietin and iron, which stimulates erythropoiesis and iron uptake by bone marrow cells and conversely draws iron from macrophages, thereby reducing cytotoxic effects [197].

A third cause of ACD results from reduced erythropoiesis activity which is due to an inadequate erythropoietin response to anemia and tissue hypoxia [68, 128, 184]. In contrast to renal anemia this is not an erythropoietin deficiency but rather a possibly cytokine-determined dysregulation. This means that the anemia cannot be compensated by increased erythropoietin synthesis. A functional relative erythropoietin deficiency results, which can be substituted.

In certain cases a hemolytic component also contributes to pathogenesis of anemia, for example due to autoantibodies in the context of a malignant systemic disease or an autoimmune disease.

If hemolysis or a reduced erythropoietin response is the predominant factor in the genesis of the ACD, then the anemia may be normocytic in character rather than microcytic. In the case of marked hemolysis the reticulocyte count is in the normal to elevated range. If, in contrast, iron redistribution and diminished erythropoietic activity is predominant, then a lowered reticulocyte count and microcytic anemia is to be expected.

The pathomechanisms responsible for tumor anemia or anemia of chronic disease in inflammations described above, such as downregulation of transferrin production, iron redistribution into macrophages as well as an insufficient erythropoietin response fulfill a biological purpose in the genesis of tumor anemias since fast-growing tumor cells are hereby iron-depleted which, however, contributes to anemia. The iron depletion of erythropoiesis is reflected in the elevated concentration of soluble transferrin receptor, especially in patients with concomitant iron deficiency or after administration of EPO.

Furthermore, in malignant diseases of the hematopoietic system induction of autoantibodies (e.g. cold agglutinins) and splenomegaly may contribute to increased hemolysis, which, as a long-term effect, leads to an iron overload in addition to iron redistribution.

Erythropoiesis as well as hematopoiesis in general may be reduced in all malignant diseases and hematological systemic diseases such as leukemia or lymphoma with significant bone marrow infiltration. This is the prognostically most unfavorable form of a tumor anemia in terms of

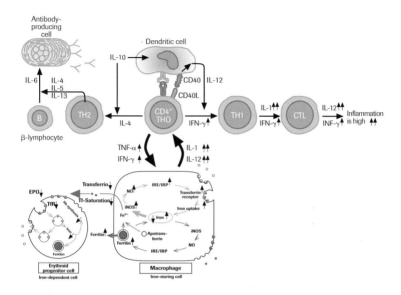

Fig. 19: Cell-cell interaction of cytokines in the differentiation of T-cells, TH1 and TH2 cells, and influence by the autoregulatory loop between iron metabolism and the NO/NOS pathway in activated macrophages.
Iron redistribution is the cause of iron overload in macrophages (tumor anemias, ACD, infections).
Moldawer, et al. (1997) [132] and Weiss, et al. (1997) [195].

responsiveness to substitution of iron and erythropoietin. This is also true for myelodysplastic syndromes in which an increased but ineffective erythropoiesis is characterized by a maximal stimulation of erythropoietin production which finally also leads to an iron overload state. These malignant bone marrow diseases can only be diagnosed adequately by bone marrow investigation performed by experts with experience in hematology.

Disturbances of Iron Utilization

Even with normal iron reserves and normal iron distribution, indicated by a normal serum ferritin concentration, disturbances of iron utilization or incorporation possibly simulate the presence of iron-deficiency anemia since they also lead to microcytic or normocytic anemia.

Ever since erythropoietin has replaced the transfusions previously used to treat renal anemia, dialysis patients have constituted the largest group. Despite adequate iron reserves, patients under erythropoietin therapy are not always able to mobilize sufficient iron from the iron stores, a situation which is shown, for example, as a reduction in transport iron (low transferritin saturation). Similarly, as in genuine iron deficiency and disturbances of iron distribution, the reduced availability of iron in heme synthesis leads to increased incorporation of zinc into the porphyrin ring. This can be measured as increased Zn-protoporphyrin in the erythrocytes, and can be used as an additional aid to the diagnosis of iron utilization disturbances with normal or elevated ferritin concentrations. Ferritin and the sTfR are suitable means of distinguishing between genuine iron deficiency and disturbances of iron distribution or utilization.

Renal Anemias

Particular attention should also be paid to iron metabolism in patients with renal anemia. The substitution of erythropoietin, together with the i.v. administration of iron, has replaced transfusions which used to be performed routinely, and has therefore revolutionized therapy.

Transfusions which previously were performed on a regular basis and the concomitant disturbance of iron utilization due to erythropoietin deficiency almost invariably led to increasing iron overload and its associated consequences. The treatment of disturbances of iron metabolism in dialysis patients is now fundamentally different since the introduction of EPO therapy, however.

The iron reserves are usually adequate, i.e. the plasma ferritin concentration is normal, or possibly increased. Despite normal iron reserves, iron mobilization is typically disturbed, which is indicated by low transferrin saturation, which can lead to relative short supply of iron in erythropoiesis and to functional iron deficiency. Generally this situation cannot be remedied by oral iron replacement therapy since in most cases, iron absorption is also disturbed.

However, as long as the erythropoietin deficiency typical of renal anemia is not corrected, the erythropoietic activity is reduced to the same extent as the iron mobilization. Therefore at a low level, iron turnover and erythropoiesis are in a steady state. Transferrin receptor expression is reduced or normal.

Renal anemia can also be complicated, for example, by a hemolytic component as a result of mechanical damage of the red cells during hemodialysis. If this is the case, a normal to elevated reticulocyte count is to be expected, and not reduced hematopoiesis, as is the case with simple erythropoietin deficiency. In this case, the short supply of iron in erythropoiesis is reflected in the elevated proportion of hypochromic erythrocytes and hypochromic reticulocytes.

However, if attempts are made to correct the erythropoietin deficiency by replacement, thereby increasing erythropoietic activity, the poor mobilization of the iron reserves is apparent as a functional iron deficiency. The cells of erythropoiesis react by increased expression of the transferrin receptor to improve iron provision. Since the ferritin concentration is generally a true reflection of the iron reserves (an exception to this is when it is immediately preceded by iron replacement or in the presence of a secondary disorder involving iron distribution disturbances) and can therefore be used as a guideline for recognizing any depot iron deficiency or for avoiding iron overload in iron replacement therapy.

Transferrin saturation is currently the best indicator of the presence of mobilized transport iron and is inversely proportional to the iron requirement. Reduced transferrin saturation in dialysis patients is a sign of inadequate iron mobilization and therefore of a functional iron deficiency requiring iron replacement (Table 3). It is possible to use the concentration of the soluble transferrin receptor as a direct indicator of the iron requirement. On no account can the transferrin receptor replace the ferritin determination for assessing the iron reserves as it only reflects the current erythropoietic activity and/or its iron requirement, which do not necessarily correlate with the iron reserves [85]. Determination of the zinc protoporphyrin in the erythrocytes has no advantage over the parameters mentioned. Because of the 120-day life-span of the erythrocytes, this determination would only reflect the iron metabolism situation at a too late stage.

Fundamentals

Table 3: Estimation of iron metabolism in dialysis patients

Iron reserves	Transport iron
Ferritin	Transferrin saturation
Generally adequate or elevated (due to transfusions, Fe replacement, disturbed Fe mobilization)	Currently best indicator for mobilizable iron
Iron absorption	**Iron requirement**
(Fe absorptiontest)	
(Generally abnormal, therefore i.v.	
Fe administration if required)	soluble transferrin receptor (sTfR)

Pathophysiology of Erythropoietin Synthesis

In progressive renal disease, erythropoietin producing cells in peritubulary capillaries lose their production capacity leading to a breakdown of the autoregulatory loop which normally guarantees a constant hemoglobin concentration [55]. In patients with renal disease this state, when combined with disturbed iron mobilization, can usually be assumed to be the cause of the anemia. Confirmation by determination of erythropoietin is necessary only in doubtful cases (Table 4).

Table 4: Erythropoietin (EPO) and ferritin concentrations in anemias and erythrocytosis

Disease	EPO concentration	Ferritin concentration
Anemias		
Iron deficiency	↑	↓
Renal anemia	↓ - ↓ ↓	n - ↑
Anemia of chronic disease	n - ↓	n - ↑ ↑
Hemolysis	↑	n - ↑
Bone marrow diseases with ineffective erythropoiesis	↑	↑ - ↑ ↑
Erythrocytosis		
Reactive in hypoxia	↑	variable
Paraneoplastic (e.g., kidney, liver carcinoma)	↑ ↑	n - ↑
Polycythemia vera	n - ↓	n - ↑

On the other hand, an insufficient erythropoietin response, probably due to cytokine effects, is probably one of the major causes of anemia of chronic disease (ACD). Absolute erythropoietin concentrations are frequently found to be within the reference range for clinically healthy persons, however this can be considered to be inadequate in patients with anemia. Inadequate erythropoietin secretion and the corresponding iron redistribution can however, be corrected by erythropoietin and iron therapy, as in renal anemia.

In contrast to these diseases (Table 4) caused by erythropoietin deficiency or insufficient response, all other anemias lead to an increased erythropoietin production as a measure of compensation. This is true for very different causes of anemia, for instance iron deficiency anemia, hemolytic anemias and many bone marrow diseases with inefficient erythropoiesis. In severe bone marrow damage (for instance aplastic anemia, myelodysplasia) this compensatory mechanism is effective no longer because the erythroid progenitor cells are missing or fail to mature.

Increased erythropoietin synthesis may lead to a secondary erythrocytosis, provided a sufficient iron supply and normal bone marrow function are present. In hypoxia (cardiopulmonary diseases, heavy smokers, high altitude) this is merely a mechanism of adaptation to oxygen deficiency. In rare cases, however, carcinomas of the kidney or the liver may produce erythropoietin which also leads to erythrocytosis [92]. In contrast to these secondary forms of erythrocytosis, polycythemia vera is an autonomous proliferation of erythroid cells which leads to a compensatory down-regulation of erythropoietin production. Determination of erythropoietin can therefore contribute to the differential diagnosis of erythrocytosis in doubtful cases.

Iron Overload

Genuine iron overload situations arise either through a biologically inappropriate increase in the absorption of iron despite adequate iron reserves, or iatrogenically as a result of frequent blood transfusions or inappropriate iron therapy.

The former condition occurs mainly as a result of the disturbance of negative feedback mechanisms, which in idiopathic hemochromatosis is manifested as a failure of the protective mechanism in the mucosa cell (see "Iron Absorption").

Conditions characterized by ineffective erythropoiesis, such as thalassemia, porphyrias, and sideroachrestic as well as hemolytic anemias - the utilization of which to synthesize hemoglobin is impaired, however - lead to increased synthesis of erythropoietin, transferrin receptor expression, and absorption of iron, despite adequate iron reserves. The iron overload in these cases is aggravated by the necessary transfusions and by the body's inability to actively excrete iron. All the mechanisms mentioned ultimately lead to overloading of the iron stores, and hence redistribution to the parenchymal cells of many organs, such as the liver, heart, pancreas, and gonads. If the storage capacity of ferritin or of the lysosomes is exceeded, the release of free iron ions and lysosomal enzymes can have a toxic effect.

The toxic effects of iron overload are due to the presence of free iron ions which are able to form oxygen radicals. The main manifestations in these organs are toxic liver damage with liver cirrhosis and primary liver cell carcinoma, heart failure, diabetes or impotence. Phagocytosis and oxidative burst of granulocytes and monocytes may be impaired as well.

Epidemiological investigations have revealed iron overload to be a risk factor for atherosclerosis, and, therefore, for coronary heart disease and cerebral sclerosis, due to increased oxidation of lipoproteins [60].

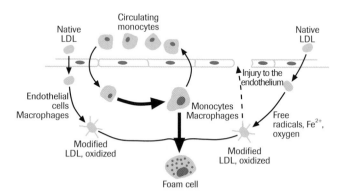

Fig. 20: The oxidation of low-density lipoprotein (LDL) and foam cell formation are promoted by iron overload states and can contribute to atherosclerosis and coronary heart disease [Steinberg, et al. (1989), 173]

This calls for an increased surveillance of iron overload in the latent phase already by regular ferritin determinations (warning limit > 400 mg/ml ferritin) and sTfR determinations. This is true not only for primary hemochromatosis or secondary hemosiderosis and hematological disease but particularly also in patients with renal anemia or anemia of chronic disease undergoing erythropoietin and iron substitution.

Almost all genuine iron overload conditions are recognizable by elevated plasma ferritin concentrations together with elevated iron levels and increased transferrin saturation values, usually with a compensating decrease in transferrin synthesis. The increased transferrin saturation, as a sign of increased iron turnover and iron transport, distinguishes iron overload from conditions with redistribution of iron and non-representatively raised plasma ferritin concentrations.

Transferrin receptor expression can vary, depending on the reason for the iron overload, in particular whether erythropoiesis is increased or decreased. Correspondingly there is also an elevated transferrin receptor concentration in the plasma in all hemolytic conditions with raised erythropoietic activity. Contrary to this, all bone marrow disorders with reduced erythropoiesis such as aplastic anemia and renal failure (without erythropoietin therapy) are characterized by reduced transferrin receptor expression. Erythropoiesis is not directly affected in hemochromatosis. Transferrin receptor expression may be normal or decreased.

Primary Hemochromatosis

Primary hemochromatosis represents the most important form of hereditary iron overload. Until now its significance has been underestimated. Nevertheless, a close association between primary hemochromatosis and certain HLA patterns has been known for quite some time. Recently, two mutations of the HLA-H gene or the HFE gene were discovered and have been found in the majority of hemochromatosis patients in the homozygous or complementary heterozygous form. The cys-282-tyr mutation is by far the most common mutation and is present in homozygous form in almost 100% of Scandinavian hemochromatosis patients and as many as 69% of Italian hemochromatosis patients. The less common variant is the his-63-asp mutation. Hemochromatoses probably represent the most common of all genetic defects. In the Caucasian population the frequency of the heterozygous defect is 1:15 and that of the homozygous form 1:200 to 1:300.

The mutations obviously give rise to an abnormal HFE protein in the epithelial cells of the mucosa of the small intestine in the region that is relevant for iron absorption. It has been known for quite some time that an inadequately elevated iron resorption represents a major patho-mechanism in the development of hemochromatosis. Mutated HFE proteins apparently lead to an inadequately elevated iron absorption and therefore to a failure of the protective mechanism in mucosal cells by a failure to inhibit the transferrin receptor (see "Iron Absorption").

Not all patients who have a homozygous gene defect actually develop manifest hemochromatosis. The frequency of hemochromatosis in the Caucasian population is in the order of 1:1000 to 1:2000. This is probably primarily due to the fact that the precondition for clinical manifestation of hemochromatosis is iron overloading of approximately 10-20 g corresponding to serum ferritin values of approximately 1000-2000 μg/L. Assuming a positive iron balance of approximately 1 mg per day (f.i. 2 mg absorption, 1 mg excretion), the time required for the accumulation of an appropriate excess of iron reserves is approximately 30-60 years. This correlates well with the main age of manifestation in men (35-55 years of age). Although the homozygous gene defect is more commonly found in women than men as a result of an evolutionary natural selection process, these women are mostly protected from the development of hemochromatosis until at least the onset of menopause. This is due to the fact that the excess iron absorption is approximately compensated for by iron loss of the same order of magnitude (15-30 mg) in the course of menstrual bleeding. Therefore the process of iron accumulation and iron over-loading in women with homozygous hemochromatic genes only commences at the onset of menopause and (compared to the process occurring in men) is delayed by decades into old age. Accordingly, only about 10% patients with symptomatic hemochromatosis are women. In an evolutionary context this means that hemochromatic genes probably represent a natural selection advantage because they protect women against severe iron deficiency until at least the onset of menopause. Only after achievement of a significantly longer life-expectancy does iron accumulation prove to be disadvantageous. Patients with heterozygous defects accumulate increased iron stores as well, but they rarely develop clinical manifestations.

The genetic defect can now be identified in the course of routine diagnostic procedures. These days PCR detection of the appropriate mutations represents the second level in hematochromatosis diagnostics after ferritin and transferrin saturation screening. Assaying for ferritin remains the decisive determination for the monitoring of iron reserves.

Other Hereditary States of Iron Overload

New insights have been gained concerning the role of ceruloplasmin in iron metabolism. This copper transporting protein seems to be important for intracellular oxidation of Fe^{2+} to Fe^{3+} which is necessary for release of iron ions from the cells and the binding to transferrin. This is exemplified by the very rare hereditary aceruloplasminemia where the lack of iron oxidation prevents binding to transferrin and thereby leads to intracellular trapping of iron ions and consequently to the development of an iron overload which resembles hereditary hemochromatosis. However, in contrast to hemochromatosis the central nervous system is also affected. Due to the impaired transferrin binding, however, iron concentrations and transferrin saturation in plasma are low whereas ferritin concentrations are high reflecting the impaired iron distribution and release.

In subjects with "African Dietary Iron Overload" the increased dietary iron intake from excessive consumption of beer home-brewed in steel drums was long considered the only cause of this iron overload disorder resembling hemochromatosis. However, a non-HLA-linked gene has now additionally been implicated which, as in hemochromatosis, may impair the protective mechanism in the mucosal cells.

Non-iron-induced Disturbances of Erythropoiesis

Disturbances of Stem Cell Proliferation

Even at the stem-cell level, physiological cell maturation can be compromised by numerous noxae and deficiencies, which in this case leads not only to anemia, but also to disturbances of myelopoiesis and thrombocytopoiesis. Examples that can be cited are medullary aplasia induced by autoimmune (e.g., thymoma), infectious (e.g., hepatitis) or toxic (e.g., antineoplastic drugs) processes or ionizing radiation. Chemical noxae or irradiation can, however, also lead to hyperregenerative bone-marrow insufficiency (myelodysplasia, MDS = myelodysplastic syndrome) with transition to acute leukemia. Whereas the above-mentioned diseases can be adequately diagnosed only by invasive and costly bone-marrow investigations, the causes of vitamin-deficiency-induced disturbances of the proliferation and maturation of bone-marrow cells with macrocytic anemia can be detected more simply by the determination of vitamin B_{12} or folic acid in the serum.

Vitamin B_{12} and Folic Acid Deficiency Cause Hyperhomocysteinemia

Since the very low daily cobalamin requirement of about 2 µg can be easily covered with a normal, varied diet, diet-induced vitamin B_{12} deficiency is rare, except in radical vegetarians. The vast majority of deficiency syndromes are therefore caused either by a deficiency of intrinsic factor (chronic atrophic gastritis, gastric resection, antibodies to intrinsic factor) or by disturbances of absorption (fish tapeworm, intestinal diseases).

Folic acid deficiency arises mainly as a result of unbalanced diet and reduced storage in liver damage, especially in connection with alcoholism. Other important causes are malabsorption in intestinal diseases and inhibition of the folic acid synthesis of intestinal bacteria by antibacterial or cytotoxic chemotherapy with folic acid antagonists. The intracellular bioavailability of the active form of tetrahydrofolic acid also depends on an adequate supply of vitamin C (reduction) and in particular of vitamin B_{12} (intracellular uptake). On account of the transfer of C1 units, folic acid and vitamin B_{12} act synergistically in DNA synthesis and cell maturation. Deficiencies similarly lead to macrocytic anemia. On account of the reduced proliferation capacity, especially of the cells of erythropoiesis, the total count of erythrocytes is then significantly reduced. However, since the hemoglobin synthesis capacity is at the same time normal, the individual erythrocytes are not only abnormally large ("macrocytes," Fig. 22), but they are also have an elevated hemoglobin content ("hyperchromic anemia"). In view of the fact that the forms of anemia are the same and that folic acid is active only with an adequate vitamin B_{12} supply, a first diagnosis of macrocytic anemia requires the simultaneous determination of vitamin B_{12} and folic acid and, in doubtful cases, the exclusion of MDS.

If folic acid deficiency is suspected, then the serum folic acid concentration may be within the lower reference range. This can indicate a latent folic acid deficiency which can possibly be proven by determining the folic acid content of erythrocytes. If serum concentrations are normal but the erythrocytes are nevertheless supplied with an insufficient amount of folic acid, then an uptake disorder is manifest which is most often caused by a vitamin B_{12} deficiency.

As a result of new findings, latent vitamin B_{12} or folic acid deficiency have recently also received more attention. Manifestations of this latent vitamin deficiency prior to the appearance of anemia or funicular spinal disease in vitamin B_{12} deficiency can lead to other metabolic anomalies such as hyperhomocysteinemia, an elevated risk of neural tube defects, immune deficiencies and atherosclerosis. New investigations in subjects with hyperhomocysteinemia suggest that the reference interval for vitamin B_{12} and folic acid must be corrected upward.

Recently the term "metabolic vitamin B_{12} or folic acid deficiency" has been introduced. It is characterized by the presence of deficiency symptoms (predominantly macrocytic anemia) already at vitamin B_{12} or folic acid concentrations in the lower reference range, possibly due to an increased demand sometimes in the context of MDS or neoplasia. This may be confirmed by further laboratory investigations. Latent or functional folic acid deficiency leads to hyperhomocysteinemia, latent and functional vitamin B_{12} deficiency mainly to an increased concentration of methylmalonic acid and possibly also of homocysteine. Vitamin B_{12} deficiency can be considered very unlikely, however, if the serum concentration is above 300 ng/l. This is also true for folic acid concentrations within a functionally defined reference range above 4.4 ng/ml.

Hemoglobinopathies

Hemoglobinopathies are a disturbance in the synthesis of the protein components of hemoglobin. A distinction is made between point mutations with exchange of individual amino acids and defects in whole protein chains. Of the former, sickle-cell anemia is the most important because it is widespread in the black population of Africa and America. The substitution of valine for glutaminic acid as sixth amino acid in the β-chain leads to the synthesis of "sickle-cell hemoglobin" (HbS), which has a very low solubility when it is not O_2 saturated. In oxygen deficiency, the change in conformation leads to precipitation of the HbS and the appearance of the characteristic sickle-shaped red cells (drepanocytes, Fig. 22). These are visible under the microscope and can therefore be used diagnostically. Atypical sickle-cell hemoglobin can also be detected by hemoglobin electrophoresis. Recently, the PCR has been used to determine the gene defect.

Hemoglobinopathies in the broader sense also include thalassemias. The widespread immigration into Central and Northern Europe from the Mediterranean area has greatly increased the importance of these disorders, especially in pediatrics. The term refers to a condition in which

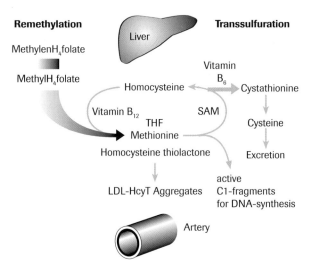

Fig. 21: **Metabolism of homocysteine, folate, vitamin B$_{12}$, vitamin B$_6$**
according to Herrmann W et al., 1997 [81]
SAM: S-Adenysyl-Methionin
THF: Tetrahydrofolate
LDL-HycT Aggregates: Low-Density-Lipoprotein-Homocysteine-
Transferase Aggregates

there is reduced synthesis or complete absence of entire chains from the hemoglobin molecule. Since α-chains are contained in fetal HbF as well as in HbA₀ and HBA₂, α-chain thalassemia has an impact on the fetus and patients of all ages. The absence of the α-chains is offset in the fetus by the formation of tetramers from γ-chains (Hbγ$_4$ = Bart's Hb), and after birth, by the formation of tetramers from β-chains (Hbβ$_4$ = Hb H). Erythrocytes with these pathological hemoglobins have a tendency to aggregate, however, and are broken down early. Since the synthesis of α-chains is coded for by 4 genes, 4 clinical pictures of varying severity can be identified, depending on the number of defective genes: a defect in one gene is manifested merely as an increased proportion of the above-mentioned pathological variants of hemoglobin, a 2-gene defect produces mild anemia, a 3-gene defect produces pronounced anemia with premature hemolysis. The complete loss of the α-chains is incompatible with the survival of the fetus.

By contrast with α-thalassemia, β-thalassemia does not have an effect until infancy or childhood when the γ-chains are replaced by β-chains. If this is not possible, HbF (with γ-chains) and HbA₂ (with δ-chains) is formed by way of compensation. Depending on its mode of inheritance, a distinction can be made between a heterozygous form (thalassemia minor) with reduced β-chain synthesis and correspondingly milder anemia, and a homozygous form (thalassemia major) with more or less complete absence of β-chains and severe anemia.

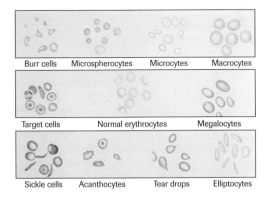

Burr cells	Microspherocytes	Microcytes	Macrocytes
Target cells	Normal erythrocytes		Megalocytes
Sickle cells	Acanthocytes	Tear drops	Elliptocytes

Fig. 22: Normal and pathological forms of erythrocytes
(modified by Diem H, according to Begemann, Rastetter (1993) [13])

The pathological variants of hemoglobin in thalassemia lead to characteristic abnormalities in the shape of erythrocytes (microcytic anemia with target cells, Fig. 22), which are detectable microscopically, whereas more precise differentiation is possible only by hemoglobin electrophoresis and the PCR, if applicable. Pathophysiologically, these structural and morphological abnormalities of erythrocytes result in more or less pronounced insufficiency as oxygen carriers and lead to an increased aggregation tendency. In addition, deformation also leads to accelerated destruction of erythrocytes, predominantly in the spleen, with all the signs of corpuscular hemolytic anemia. For signs of hemolysis and hemolytically-determined iron overload, refer to the chapter entitled "Pathologically Increased Hemolysis."

Disturbances of Porphyrin Synthesis

Disturbances of porphyrin synthesis [48] are to be considered here only in so far as they may affect erythropoiesis and lead to anemia (Fig. 23). These forms of anemia are called sideroachrestic, since the iron provided for Hb synthesis in the bone marrow cannot be used, despite adequate reserves, and is consequently stored in the erythroblasts.

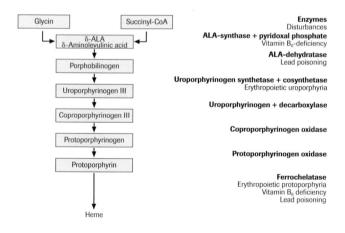

Fig. 23: Disturbances of porphyrin synthesis with possible anemia

The erythroblasts, which are thus overloaded with iron, are then termed sideroblasts, and can be detected in the bone marrow using iron-specific stains. In sideroachrestic anemia, however, the inadequately increased iron absorption results in the development of generalized, genuine iron overload over a longer period, but especially after repeated transfusions; it is recognizable from an elevated serum ferritin concentration. Most of the causes of sideroachrestic anemia are comparatively uncommon, and therefore rarely need to be considered in practice. Hereditary erythropoietic porphyrias such as congenital erythropoietic uroporphyria (Günther's disease) with a defect of uroporphyrinogen III synthase and erythropoietic protoporphyria with a defect of ferrochelatase are particularly rare. Acquired forms such as pyridoxal phosphate (vitamin B_6) deficiency are slightly more common; this may be of nutritional origin, in alcoholics, for example, or arise as a result of isoniazid therapy in tuberculosis patients, and leads to a disturbance of iron incorporation via inhibition of δ-amino-levulinic acid synthase and ferrochelatase. Similar pathological mechanisms are also at the root of lead-induced anemia and disturbance of porphyrin synthesis. Chronic lead intoxication leads to inhibition of δ-amino-levulinic acid dehydratase and of ferrochelatase. All the above-mentioned causes ultimately produce a disturbance of iron utilization via the synthesis of an incomplete porphyrin skeleton or via the direct inhibition of ferrochelatase, with the general features of sideroachrestic (sideroblastic) anemia described above. If the defect is mainly in the terminal stage of the reaction (incorporation of iron by ferrochelatase), zinc is incorporated into the finished protoporphyrin skeleton instead of iron, recognizable from the increased concentration of Zn-protoporphyrin in the erythrocytes. Defects at earlier stages in porphyrin synthesis can be identified by analysis of the corresponding intermediate products; lead and vitamin B_6 can also be determined directly for confirmation of the diagnosis. A disturbance of iron utilization at the mitochondrial level yet to be explained is also found in patients with myelodysplastic syndrome (MDS).

Pathologically Increased Hemolysis

"Hemolysis" is the term generally used in clinical medicine to describe the pathologically increased or premature destruction of erythrocytes.

The cause of this may lie in structural or biochemical defects in the erythrocytes themselves ("corpuscular hemolysis"), in which case it takes place mainly in the macrophages of the RES in the spleen or the liver. By contrast, extracorpuscular hemolysis takes place mainly intravascularly through the action of autoantibodies, toxins, infective organisms or physical noxae, such as artificial heart valves. Intravascular hemolysis can be detected very sensitively by means of clinical chemistry investigations, since hemoglobin and erythrocyte enzymes, e.g. LDH isoenzymes 1 and 2, pass into the peripheral blood even at a low hemolysis rate.

Haptoglobin

Since free hemoglobin is rapidly bound to α_2-haptoglobin and this hemoglobin-haptoglobin complex is also rapidly phagocytized by the RES, a selective reduction in free haptoglobin is regarded as the most sensitive sign of intravascular hemolysis which at the same time also has a high degree of diagnostic specificity [135]. The only other possible causes are severe protein-loss syndromes or disturbances of protein synthesis. This applies in particular to advanced liver diseases (e.g. liver cirrhosis) with a severe synthesis defect which also includes haptoglobin. A reduction in haptoglobin may also be produced, albeit less commonly, by gastrointestinal protein-loss syndromes which also non-selectively include macromolecular proteins, such as celiac disease and Whipple's disease. Since haptoglobin also serves as a proteinase inhibitor, its synthesis in the liver is increased during acute-phase reactions. The resultant increase in concentration may then "mask" any hemolysis which is present simultaneously (Tab. 5).

Table 5: Differentiation: Hemolysis, acute-phase reaction and protein loss or disturbance of protein synthesis

Disease	Haptoglobin	Hemopexin	CRP
Mild Hemolysis	↓ - ↓ ↓	n	n
Severe Hemolysis	↓ ↓	↓	n
Hemolysis and acute-phase reaction	n - ↑	n - ↓	↑ ↑
Acute-phase reaction	↑ - ↑ ↑	n	↑ ↑
Nephrotic syndrome	↑ - ↑ ↑	↓	n - ↓
Gastrointestinal protein loss or disturbance of protein synthesis	↓	↓	n - ↓

Features of Severe Hemolysis

Free hemoglobin occurs in the plasma only if the hemoglobin binding capacity of haptoglobin is exceeded; if the renal threshold is exceeded, excretion in the urine is also possible. Excess heme can also be bound in the blood by hemopexin and be removed from the plasma in the form of a heme-hemopexin complex. Hemoglobinuria and a reduction in serum hemopexin are thus signs of severe hemolysis.

In addition to the changes described, increased amounts of LDH isoenzymes 1 and 2 are released from the erythrocytes into plasma. The degradation of heme leads, independently of the site of the hemolytic process, to an increased amount of unconjugated bilirubin and of iron. Because of the simultaneous inappropriately increased iron absorption and the possible need for transfusions, all chronic forms of hemolysis are associated with iron overload, recognizable as an increased serum ferritin concentration. With adequate bone marrow function, increased hemolysis, especially extracorpuscular forms, can be compensated for by new formation which can be boosted up to 10-fold. This is shown as an increased passage of immature erythrocytes (reticulocytes) into the peripheral blood. Anemia develops only if the hemolysis rate exceeds the bone marrow capacity. Due to the larger volume of reticulocytes, the anemia can be macrocytic.

If, in the long run, the binding capacity of haptoglobin and hemopexin is exceeded during severe intravascular hemolysis and, as a consequence of this, larger amounts of free hemoglobin are filtered through the glomeruli and therefore excreted, then the hemolysis may lead to iron deficiency in individual cases because of the chronic loss of iron. If, however, iron loss does not occur in this manner, then iron overload is usually the consequence of chronic hemolysis as described above. This can be differentiated by regular urine investigations and ferritin determinations in serum.

Causes of Hemolysis (Corpuscular, Extracorpuscular)

Corpuscular hemolysis can also be induced by defects in the erythrocyte membrane, in addition to the hemoglobinopathies such as sickle-cell anemia or thalassemia mentioned earlier. The most important example of such a membrane defect is spherocytic anemia (hereditary sphero-cytosis) which can be diagnosed on the basis of characteristic morpho-logical changes ("microspherocytes") (Fig. 23) and the reduced osmo-tic resistance of the erythrocytes. Other causes are defects of erythrocyte enzymes which are required for the stabilization of functionally impor-tant proteins, e.g. glucose-6-phosphatedehydrogenase deficiency. While this disease has also become important in Central and Northern Europe as a result of immigration from the Mediterranean area, all other defects of erythrocyte enzymes are definitely rarities. The most important ac-quired form of corpuscular hemolysis is PNH (paroxsymal nocturnal hemoglobinuria) (Tab. 6).

Numerous noxae most of which can be identified from the case history or by means of simple laboratory investigations produce intra-vascular hemolysis by directly damaging the erythrocytes themselves; these include mechanical hemolysis after heart valve replacement or in the case of microangiopathies (Burr cells) toxins such as snake venoms or detergents; other causes include infective organisms such as malarial plasmodia, or hemolysis as a consequence of gram-negative sepsis. Intra-vascular hemolysis can be identified independently of the causes on the basis of the above-mentioned general features of hemolysis. However, in the case of the autoimmune hemolytic anemias, which can occur in the context of autoimmune diseases, immune defects, viral infections, lymphatic malignancies and as drug-induced anemias, the causes are often difficult to determine in the individual case. A distinction is made between warm, cold and bithermal (Donath-Landsteiner) antibodies; binding of the antibodies to the patient's erythrocytes can be detected in the direct anti-human globulin test (Coombs' test). If the result is positive, further differentiation using other methods is necessary.

Table 6: Diagnosis of corpuscular hemolytic anemias

Disease	Erythrocyte forms	Confirmation test
Hereditary spherocytosis	Micro spherocytes	Osmotic resistance
Thalassemia	Target cells	Hemoglobin electrophoresis, PCR
Sickle cell anemia	Sickle cells	Hemoglobin electrophoresis, PCR
Erythrocyte enzyme defects unspecific (e. G. Gluc-6-PD-deficiency)	Heinz Bodies	Erythrocyte enzymes
PNH (paroxysmal nocturnal hemoglobi-nuria or Marchiafava-Micheli Syndrome)	unspecific	Defect of glycolipid anchor antigens such as CD59 and CD55

GLU-6-PO = glucose-6-phosphate dehydrogenase deficiency; PCR = polymerase chain reaction, CD = cluster of differentiation

Diagnosis of Disturbances of Iron Metabolism
Disturbances of Erythropoiesis

Life-threatening clinical states are very rare occurrences in the majority of anemia diagnoses. An important component of therapy, therefore, is to determine the cause of the anemia, classify it, and eliminate it in a subsequent step.

In the majority of cases, disturbances of iron metabolism are triggered by disturbances in the body's iron balance which, in turn, is controlled entirely by absorption. The uptake of iron therefore occupies the key position in the iron metabolism as a whole (Fig. 24). The daily iron requirement depends on age and sex. It is increased in puberty and in pregnancy. The total iron pool is more or less constant in adults. The quantity of iron absorbed is about 10% (1 mg) of the quantity consumed daily in the normal diet, but this fraction can increase to 2 to 4 mg in conditions of iron deficiency.

Physiological loss of iron is low, and it is comparable to the quantity absorbed. It takes place as a result of the shedding of intestinal epithelial cells and through excretion in bile, urine and perspiration.

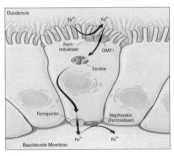

Fig. 24: Iron transport through the intestinal epithelial cells. Iron must be transported through two membranes in order to travel from the lumen of the bowels into the baso-lateral space. The transport protein that channels Fe^{2+} through the cell membrane is DMT1 (divalent metal transporter 1). Fe^{3+} is reduced by a ferric reductase. Fe^{3+} is transported through the baso-lateral membrane by ferroportin. Fe^{2+} is oxidized to Fe^{3+} by a protein related to ceruloplasmin (ferroxidase; hephaestin). According to N. C. Andrews (1999) [4]

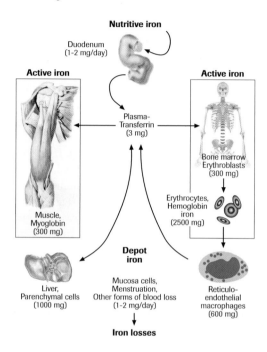

Fig. 25: Active iron, transport iron, iron stores in iron metabolism.
According to N. C. Andrews (1999) [4]

Since the absorption and the loss of iron are limited under physiological conditions, the quantity of storage iron can only be increased by massive supplies from outside the body. Every transfusion of one liter of blood increases the quantity of storage iron in the body by about 250 mg.

Disturbances in iron absorption can be detected by an iron absorption test. After collecting a blood sample from a fasting patient to determine the baseline value for the serum iron concentration, approximately 200 mg of a bivalent iron preparation is administered. A second blood collection is performed after 3 hours. With normal iron absorption, there should be an increase to 2-3 times the baseline value during the observation period.

A reduced or delayed rise indicates a disturbance of iron absorption. An increased rise is found in rare forms of iron deficiency, and in primary hemochromatosis [200].

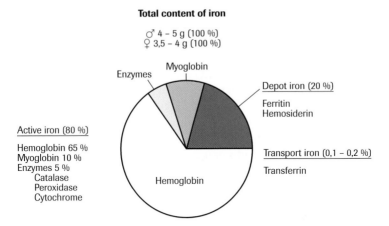

Total content of iron

♂ 4 – 5 g (100 %)
♀ 3,5 – 4 g (100 %)

Enzymes

Myoglobin

Depot iron (20 %)

Ferritin
Hemosiderin

Active iron (80 %)

Hemoglobin 65 %
Myoglobin 10 %
Enzymes 5 %
Catalase
Peroxidase
Cytochrome

Transport iron (0,1 – 0,2 %)

Transferrin

Hemoglobin

Fig. 26: Total content of iron in the body

Excess iron that is not used for the synthesis of hemoglobin, myoglobin, or iron enzymes is stored in the depot proteins ferritin and hemosiderin.

The total iron content of the healthy human body is about 3.5 to 4 g in women and 4 to 5 g in men [151]. About 70% of this is stored in hemoglobin, 10% is contained in iron-containing enzymes and myoglobin, 20% in the body's iron depot, and only 0.1 to 0.2% is bound to transferrin as transport iron (Fig. 26). However, this distribution applies only under optimum nutritional conditions.

Hemoglobin accounts for approximately 80% of the active iron.

One gram of hemoglobin is equal to 3.4 mg iron.

Since the life cycle of the red blood cells is 120 days, an adult requires about 16 to 20 mg of iron daily in order to replace these vital cells [22]. Most of the iron required for this purpose comes by lysed red blood cells. During pregnancy and breast-feeding, the additional iron requirement is far in excess of the quantity of absorbable iron contained in the food. The loss of iron in normal menstruation is about 15 to 30 mg (100 ml of blood contains about 50 mg of iron). The additional iron requirement during pregnancy is between 700 and 1000 mg.

Clinical Aspects

As a result of menstruation and pregnancy, the quantity of depot iron in women decreases through blood loss to 250 mg, i.e. only 5 to 10% of the total iron content. According to a WHO estimate, 50% of all fertile women in western countries suffer from hypoferremia.

The second largest component in active iron is myoglobin, at about 10%. Like hemoglobin, myoglobin is an oxygen-binding hemoprotein with a molecular weight of about 17,100 daltons. It is formed in the striated muscle (skeletal muscle and myocardium). Because it has a higher affinity for oxygen than hemoglobin, myoglobin is responsible for the transportation and storage of oxygen in the striated muscles. The diagnostic specificity of the serum myoglobin determination is limited, since it is not possible to differentiate between skeletal muscle myoglobin and myocardium myoglobin. An increase in the serum is observed in all forms of muscle disease and injuries, and in myocardial infarction. The diagnostic value in the assessment of impaired kidney function is limited, since myoglobin is degraded to monomers and is completely eliminated with the urine. The determination of myoglobin in sports medicine for the assessment of performance is worthy of mention.

Case History and Clinical Findings

According to WHO criteria (World Health Organization. Nutritional anemias. Series 1992: 503), anemia exists when the concentration of hemoglobin falls below the following values:

Table 7: Criteria for anemia

		Hemoglobin [g/dL]
Adults	Men	13.5
	Women(< 50 years of age)	12.5
	Women(> 50 years of age)	13.5
Children	(< 16 years of age)	11.5

Anemia is caused by the following, for example:
- Deficiency of iron or vitamin B_{12}, vitamin B_6, folate
- Chronic disturbances of distribution, chronic inflammation
- Anemias of infection
- Tumor anemias
- Chronic disturbances of utilization, uremic anemias
- Blood loss
- Erythrocytic decomposition (hemolysis)
- Impaired erythrocyte formation (toxic or neoplastic processes)
- Iron overoad (hemochromatosis)

Table 8: Case history and clinical findings in patients with anemia

Case history:	• Genetic hemolytic disturbances
	• Dizziness, shortness of breath, paleness, icterus
	• Unusual stools
	• History of gynecological bleeding
	• Eating and drinking habits (iron deficiency in vegetarians, vitamin B_{12} deficiency, alcoholism)
	• Hemolysis and aplasia induced by medication
Clinical findings:	• Advanced anemia: Fatigue, shortness of breath, dizziness
	• Additional iron deficiency: (angular stomatitis, brittle nails, brittle hair)
	• Hemolysis Flu-like symptoms with discoloration of sclera, skin and urine, occasional splenodynia, ostalgia)
	• Vitamin B_{12} deficiency: Subicteric colorite, inflammation of the tongue, occasional signs of bleeding combined with thrombocytopenia, occasional paresthesia
	• Macrocytic anemias in patients with chronic liver disease (alcohol-related and non-alcohol-related)

Clinical Aspects

The following laboratory parameters in particular have become significant and enjoy widespread application:

- *Biochemical parameters:* Determination of serum proteins and vitamin deficiency diagnostics, ferritin (iron deficiency), transferrin, transferrin saturation (iron overload), soluble transferrin receptor (disturbances of distribution and utilization), C-reactive protein (inflammations), ceruloplasmin (redistribution), haptoglobin (increased turnover), B_{12}/B_6/folate (deficiencies)
- *Hematological parameters:* Hematological blood cell count. Hemoglobin, hematocrit, red blood count (RBC), mean cell volume of erythrocytes (MCV), mean cell hemoglobin content of erythrocytes (MCH), reticulocyte count, reticulocyte index, mean cellular hemoglobin content of reticulocytes (CHr), reticulocyte production index (RPI).

The serum proteins ferritin, soluble transferrin receptor (sTfR) and C-reactive protein (CRP) are parameters with high sensitivity and specificity. The erythrocyte indices MCV, MCH, and the reticulocyte indices have found widespread use in the blood cell count of anemia diagnostics.

Clinical Significance of the Determination of Ferritin

The concentration of ferritin in the serum or plasma reflects the total body iron stores.

Ferritin is the most important iron storage protein. Together with the quantitatively and biologically less important hemosiderin, it contains about 15 to 20% of all the iron in the body. Ferritin occurs in nearly all organs. Particularly high concentrations are found in liver, spleen, and bone marrow.

A direct correlation is found for healthy adults between the plasma ferritin concentration and the quantity of available iron stored in the body. Comparative studies with quantitative phlebotomies and the histochemical assessment of bone marrow aspirates have shown that in iron deficiency and in primary or secondary stages of iron overload ferritin provides accurate information on the iron reserves available to the body for hemoglobin synthesis [97].

If more iron is supplied than the body can store as ferritin, iron is deposited as hemosiderin in the cells of the reticuloendothelial system. Unlike ferritin, hemosiderin is insoluble in water, and it is only with difficulty that its iron content can be mobilized.

Ferritin, the iron storage protein, is formed in cells in response to the intracellular iron concentration. If the intracellular iron concentration is high, a large amount of ferritin is synthesized. If the intracellular iron concentration is low, a small amount of ferritin is synthesized. A small amount of the ferritin produced is secreted by the cells into the bloodstream. A direct correlation exists when serum ferritin concentration is in the range of 12 to 200 µg/L.

---

1 ng/mL = 1 µg/L serum ferritin corresponds to 10 mg stored iron.

Serum ferritin is a good indicator of storage iron reserves, but it provides no information about the functional compartment, i.e., the amount of iron actually available for erythropoiesis, for example. A low ferritin value merely indicates that the patient is at risk of developing active iron deficiency. Normal or elevated serum ferritin values can occur in patients with active iron deficiency. This is the case, for example, with infections, acute or chronic inflammation and malignant tumors. This is due to the fact that ferritin is an acute-phase protein, the synthesis of which is increased in the states described above. The result is a disproportion-al increase in serum ferritin in relation to the storage iron reserves. In patients with ferritin values in the reference range accompanied by elevated CRP - the best indicator of an acute-phase reaction - a storage iron deficiency cannot be ruled out. Diseases and conditions in which the serum ferritin level does not reflect the content of storage iron are listed in Table 9.

The value of ferritin determination in serum/plasma was demonstrated more than 10 years ago in a comparison of the various parameters available for the determination of the body's iron stores. These results were recently confirmed [126] (Tab. 9).

Table 9: Limits of ferritin determination in the assessment of iron deficiency

- Indirect information only regarding the supply of erythropoiesis with iron

- No indication of the severity of iron deficiency in the case of low or borderline low serum ferritin values, especially in young children, adolescents in a growth spurt, serious athletes, blood donors, pregnant women

- Disproportional increase in serum ferritin in relation to reserves of storage iron in patients with:
  - Infections, acute and chronic inflammation, malignant tumors
  - Damage of the liver parenchyma, e.g., viral or alcoholic acute and chronic hepatitides, liver cirrhosis
  - Dialysis patients
  - Myelodysplastic syndrome (MDS)
  - Parenteral iron administration

Table 10: Merits of the various parameters for the detection of iron deficiency

	Sensitivity in %	Specificity in %
Serum iron +	84	43
Transferrin	84	63
Serum ferritin	79	96
Serum iron + Serum ferritin	84	42
Transferrin + Serum ferritin	84	50
Soluble transferrin receptor	92	84

Ferritin is well suited for assessment of the iron metabolism of a patient population having no primary consumptive disease or chronic inflammation. The determination of ferritin is particularly useful in the diagnosis of disturbances of iron metabolism, in the monitoring of iron therapy, for the determination of iron reserves in high-risk groups, and in the differential diagnosis of anemias [112] (Tab. 11).

Table 11: Clinical significance of ferritin

1. Representative result
   Detection of prelatent and latent iron deficiency
   Differential diagnosis of anemias
   Monitoring of high-risk groups
   Monitoring of iron therapy (oral)
   Determination of the iron status of dialysis patients and patients who have
   received multiple blood transfusions
   Diagnosis of iron overload
   Monitoring of phlebotomy therapy or chelating agent therapy

2. Non-representative result
   Destruction of hepatocellular tissue
   Infections
   Inflammations (collagen diseases)
   Malignancies
   Iron therapy (parenteral)

In clinical practice, the ferritin concentration reflects the size of the iron stores, especially at the beginning of therapy. A deficiency in the stores of the reticuloendothelial system (RES) can be detected at a particularly early stage. A value of 20 ng/ml has been found to be a suitable clinical limit for prelatent iron deficiency. A value below this reliably indicates exhaustion of the iron reserves that can be mobilized for hemoglobin synthesis. A decrease to less than 12 ng/ml is defined as latent iron deficiency. Neither of these values calls for further laboratory confirmation, even where the blood count is still morphologically normal. They are indications for therapy, though it is still necessary to look for the cause of the iron deficiency. If the reduced ferritin concentration is accompanied by hypochromic microcytic anemia, the patient is suffering from manifest iron deficiency (Tab. 12).

If the ferritin level is elevated and a disturbance of iron distribution can be ruled out by determination of the soluble transferrin receptor (sTfR) or transferrin saturation and/or of the C-reactive protein and by investigation of the blood sedimentation rate and the blood count, the raised ferritin level indicates that the body is overloaded with iron. A ferritin value of 400 ng/ml is taken as a limit. The transferrin saturation is massively increased (over 45%) in these cases.

If there is no evidence of any other disease, primary or secondary hemochromatosis must be suspected. Differential diagnosis must be pursued through history-taking, molecular biological detection, possibly supplemented with a liver biopsy, bone-marrow puncture, or MRI. Diagnosis of a primary hemochromatosis calls for further investigations for organic lesions.

Raised ferritin values are ambiguous, and are found in a number of inflammatory diseases, in the presence of malignant growths, and in the presence of damage to the liver parenchyma. Elevated ferritin levels are also found in a number of anemias arising from various causes in some cases with true iron overload. Recent oral or, in particular, parenteral iron therapy can also lead to raised non-representative ferritin values.

These increases in the ferritin concentration are generally due to disturbances of distribution, and differential diagnosis is possible by determination of the transferrin concentration and of the transferrin saturation. In all these processes, the transferrin value is reduced or close to the lower limit of the reference range (< 200 mg/dL). The transferrin saturation is low to normal (< 15%), and hypochromic anemia can often be diagnosed on the basis of the blood count.

Table 12: Ferritin concentrations in healthy individuals and in patients with iron deficiency and iron overload [75]

Reference range in men and women over 50 years of age	30-400 ng/mL = 30-400 µg/L
Reference range in women under 50 years of age	15-150 ng/mL = 15-150 µg/L
Prelatent iron deficiency (storage iron deficiency)	< 20 ng/mL
Latent and manifest iron deficiency (iron deficiency anemia)	< 12 ng/mL
Representative iron overload	> 400 ng/mL

Transferrin, Transferrin Saturation

Transferrin is synthesized in the liver and is controlled by the iron content in the hepatocyte. In healthy individuals, 15 to 45% of transferrin is saturated with iron. When the iron supply of the functional compartment is inadequate, transferrin synthesis is increased by way of compensation, which leads to a decrease in transferrin saturation. In the presence of infections, acute or chronic inflammation and malignant tumors, transferrin synthesis is down-regulated regardless of the status of active iron. For this reason, transferrin saturation is not an indicator of iron supply of the functional compartment and cannot be used in any anemia accompanied by an increase in CRP. Conditions and diseases in which the transferrin saturation does not provide relevant results for diagnosing iron deficiency are listed in Tables 13 and 14.

Table 13: Transferrin in the differential diagnosis of disturbances or iron metabolism

1. *Normal to slightly reduced transferrin concentrations*
   Primary hemochromatosis (exception: late stage secondary hemochromatosis)

2. *Decreased transferrin concentrations*
   Infections
   Inflammations/collagen diseases
   Malignant tumors
   Hemodialysis patients
   Cirrhosis of the liver-Disturbances of synthesis
   Nephrotic syndrome-Losses
   Ineffective erythropoiesis
   (e.g. sideroachrestic and megaloblastic anemias)
   Thalassemias

3. *Increased transferrin concentrations*
   Iron deficiency
   Estrogen-induced increase in synthesis (pregnancy, medication)
   Ineffective erythropoiesis (some forms, e.g. myelodysplastic syndromes)

Table 14: Disadvantages of the transferrin saturation for assessing iron deficiency

- Transferrin is an anti-acute-phase protein, the synthesis of which is reduced in the presence of infections, inflammation and malignant tumors regardless of iron supply. A reduced serum concentration results.

- Transferrin is released in the presence of hepatocellular damage, resulting in a serum concentration that is inadequately high for iron supply.

- Pregnancy and estrogen therapy increase transferrin synthesis. The serum concentration is not an indicator of iron supply.

- The transferrin saturation is higher than before, even hours after eating.

- The transferrin saturation does not drop below 15% until hemoglobin decreases to 2 g/dL below the baseline value when the storage iron reserves are empty.

Clinical Aspects

Elevated transferrin values are found in the presence of iron deficiency and particularly in pregnancy. The transferrin level may also be raised as a result of drug induction (administration of oral contraceptives). A detailed patient history is essential.

A number of rare anemias with hyperferritinemia and low transferrin levels belong to the group of sideroachrestic diseases and are congenital hypochromic microcytic anemias (atransferrinemia, antitransferrin antibodies, receptor defects).

Increased ferritin concentrations together with low transferrin levels point to anemias with ineffective erythropoiesis (thalassemias, megaloblastic, sideroblastic, and dyserythropoietic anemias). Myelodysplastic syndromes, on the other hand, may be accompanied by elevated values for both transferrin and ferritin.

Elevated ferritin concentrations unrelated to the iron stores are often found in patients with malignancies. Possible reasons that have been suggested for this phenomenon are increased ferritin synthesis by neoplastic cells, release of ferritin on decomposition of neoplastic tissue, and blockage of erythropoiesis as a result of chronic inflammatory processes in and around the tumor tissue. Ferritin determinations on patients with malignant tumors sometimes also record high concentrations of acidic isoferritins [112, 114]. In the presence of inflammations, infectious diseases, or malignant tumors, low transferrin concentrations and low transferrin saturation values point to disturbances of iron distribution. Low transferrin concentrations may be caused either by losses (renal, intestinal) or by reduced synthesis (compensation, liver damage).

Low transferrin values found for patients with cirrhosis of the liver are usually due to the defective protein metabolism. In nephrotic syndrome, so much transferrin is lost via the urine that low transferrin levels are the rule. The excretion of transferrin in the urine is used to determine the selectivity of proteinuria.

The transferrin concentration and the transferrin saturation are valuable aids in the differential diagnosis of raised ferritin concentrations. True iron overload is accompanied by increased transferrin saturation. Non-representative ferritin elevation in patients with disturbances of distribution is characterized by low transferrin saturation and low transferrin concentrations.

Soluble Transferrin Receptor (sTfR)

Transferrin receptors (TfR) are components of the cytoplasmic membrane of all cells, with the exception of erythrocytes. Approximately 75% of the transferrin receptors are located on the erythropoietic precursor cells, which have a 10 to 100-fold higher TfR content than other tissue. The function of cellular TfR is to bind two transferrin molecules, each of which is loaded with two iron atoms, and transport them via endocytosis into the cytoplasma (Fig. 12).

The number of transferrin receptors of erythropoiesis increases:

• If the iron supply of the functional compartment is inadequate. In this case, the erythropoietic precursor cells excrete more TfR.

• In the presence of disease and conditions accompanied by an increase in the mass of erythropoietic precursor cells in the bone marrow, e.g., in the presence of hemolytic anemia. Conditions such as these are identified by an increase in reticulocyte count and the reticulocyte index.

The soluble transferrin receptor (sTfR) is the form of the TfR passed into the bloodstream after proteolytic cleavage from the cytoplasmic membrane. The serum concentration of the sTfR behaves proportionally to the erythropoietic expression of the membrane-bound TfR and depends only on the iron supply of erythropoiesis when the reticulocyte index is normal. As the iron supply decreases, the serum concentration of the sTfR increases continuously. The sTfR is the only biochemical marker that indicates an inadequate iron supply of erythropoiesis. The determination of the sTfR is a valuable supplement to ferritin. Since the determination of ferritin has not yet been standardized and is offered by over 30 manufacturers around the world, there is no generally valid and accepted limit value below which a storage iron deficiency clearly exists. Limit values of 12 to 45 mg/L are cited in the literature. The determination of the sTfR as a supplement to serum ferritin is significant in individuals known to have limited storage iron, e.g., young children, adolescents in a growth spurt, serious athletes, blood donors and pregnant women.

The concentration of the sTfR in serum remains unaffected by an acute-phase reaction, so that the sTfR also indicates an active iron deficiency in the presence of infection, acute or chronic inflammation and malignant tumors. This does not apply in every case, because the level of the sTfR value is a summation of the iron deficiency-induced TfR portion and the erythropoietically proliferative portion. The latter is greatly reduced, however, since erythropoiesis is hypoproliferative in the presence of tumor anemias and anemias of chronic diseases in inflammations. In the presence of these forms of anemia, sTfR concentrations that exceed the upper reference range value are not reached in more than 50% of cases, despite the iron deficiency.

Iron deficiency, regardless of the cause, leads to an increased expression of the transferrin receptor and, accordingly, to an increased concentration of the soluble transferrin receptor in the plasma. All forms of storage iron deficiency can be detected with a great deal of certainty by a low concentration of ferritin in the plasma. Measuring the soluble transferrin receptor therefore does not offer an advantage in this case. In cases with adequate iron reserves coupled with functional iron deficiency, i.e., disturbances of iron utilization, an increased concentration of the soluble transferrin receptor indicates inadequate supply of iron to erythropoiesis or inadequate iron mobilization [186].

Patients with *malignant neoplasias and chronic inflammation* develop a deficiency of transport and active iron accompanied by a simultaneous relative overloading of the iron stores and a simultaneous relative inadequate supply of iron to the erythropoietic cells (as a consequence of reduced transferrin synthesis, among other things). The reduced availability of iron is a protective mechanism as well as one of the major pathomechanisms in ACD. When the disturbance of iron distribution is pronounced, the presence of a hypochromic anemia can be assumed. It can be distinguished from iron deficiency anemia by ferritin determination. In addition to reduced transferrin synthesis, an increased release of cytokines such as IFN-γ and TNF-α leads to an increased iron uptake in macrophages by means of an increased transferrin receptor expression. In the presence of ACD and tumors, this increased iron storage in macrophages also withdraws a portion of the iron from transferrin, which is already reduced. A further cause for the development of anemia is the reduced erythropoietic activity. This is definitely not due to an erythropoietin deficiency but rather a possible disturbed regulation induced by cytokines. In the majority of cases of disturbed iron distribution, an inadequate supply of iron to the erythropoietic cells coupled with a reduced erythropoietic activity is present. Accordingly, the transferrin receptor expression is usually normal.

Disturbances of iron utilization and incorporation that simulate the clinical picture of an iron deficiency anemia are also possible in the presence of *normal iron reserves* and normal iron distribution indicated by the presence of a normal serum ferritin concentration since they can also lead to a microcytic anemia. Since erythropoietin has replaced formerly-common transfusions used to treat renal anemias, dialysis patients now represent the largest group of individuals with this type of anemia [69, 167].

The ferritin concentration is generally a true reflection of the iron reserves (an exception to this is when it is immediately preceded by iron replacement or in the presence of a secondary disorder involving iron distribution disturbances) and can therefore be used as a guideline for recognizing any depot iron deficiency or for avoiding iron overload in iron replacement therapy. Transferrin saturation is currently the best indicator of the presence of mobilized transport iron and is inversely proportional to the iron requirement. Reduced transferrin saturation in dialysis patients is a sign of inadequate iron mobilization and therefore of a functional iron deficiency requiring iron replacement. It may be possible in the future to use the concentration of the soluble transferrin receptor as a direct indicator of the iron requirement. On no account can the transferrin receptor replace the ferritin determination for assessing the iron reserves as it only reflects the current erythropoietic activity and/or its iron requirement, which do not necessarily correlate with the iron reserves.

All *iron overload states* can be detected using clinical chemistry methods based on the elevated plasma ferritin concentration, the simultaneously elevated iron level and the increased transferrin saturation in the presence of transferrin synthesis that is usually reduced by way of compensation. Depending on the cause of iron overload, the transferrin receptor expression can be very different depending on whether the erythropoiesis is increased or reduced. Accordingly, an elevated concentration of the transferrin receptor in the plasma is also found in the presence of all hemolytic states with an erythropoietic activity that is increased by way of compensation. In patients with renal insufficiency (without EPO therapy), a reduced transferrin receptor expression corresponding to a greatly reduced erythropoiesis is found. Erythropoiesis is not immediately affected in the presence of hemochromatosis. Transferrin receptor expression can be normal or reduced [147].

Laboratory Diagnostics in the Case of Suspected Disturbances of Iron Metabolism

The following steps are recommended in the diagnosis of disturbances or iron metabolism (Fig. 27) [182, 183, 184]:
- Blood count to identify an anemia. An anemia exists when the hemoglobin concentration falls below the following values:

Men and women over 50 years of age	13.5 g/dL
Women under 50 years of age	12.5 g/dL
Children	11.5 g/dL

- Ferritin in the serum to assess the storage iron reserves. An iron deficiency exists and oral iron replacement is indicated when the serum ferritin values fall below the following values:

Men and women over 50 years of age	30 µg/L
Women under 50 years of age and children	15 µg/L

Range of uncertainty if an acute-phase reaction exists at the same time:

Men and women over 50 years of age	30 - 100 µg/L
Women under 50 years of age and children	15 - 100 µg/L

- CRP in the serum to determine if an inflammatory reaction influences the ferritin value. Iron deficiency is not present if CRP is < 5 mg/L with ferritin values of 30 - 100 µg/L in women over 50 years of age and in men, and in the presence of ferritin values of 15 to 100 µg/L in women under 50 years of age and in children. If the CRP level is greater than 5 mg/L, the ferritin value can be inadequately high in relation to the storage iron reserves. For this reason, ferritin values in the range of 15 (30) - 100 µg/L provide no information about iron supply.

Clinical Aspects

• STfR in serum to assess the iron supply of erythropoiesis.
- If the concentration is normal, no findings can be made, because the sTfR concentration can be in the reference range in the presence of ACD and tumor anemia due to hypoproliferative erythropoiesis, despite an iron deficiency.
- If the concentration is elevated, the iron supply of erythropoiesis is inadequate if the corrected reticulocyte index is normal. An elevated sTfR value indicates the presence of an inadequate iron supply. Oral iron replacement is indicated.

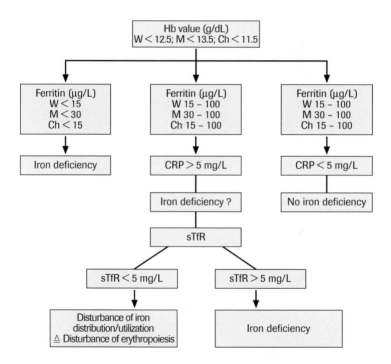

Fig. 27: Successive diagnostics in cases of suspected disturbances of iron metabolism (W = women, M = men, Ch = children)

Using mathematical relationships between three independent parameters, the laboratory diagnostics of the main disturbances of iron metabolism can be supported using a software program (Fig. 28).

The following independent parameters are used:
- Ferritin, as an analyte with which the current total content of iron in the body (depot iron) can be estimated,
- STfR, as an analyte with which the erythropoietic activity (active iron) can be estimated,
- CRP, as an analyte that is used to diagnose non-specific disturbances of iron metabolism caused by inflammatory processes, for example.

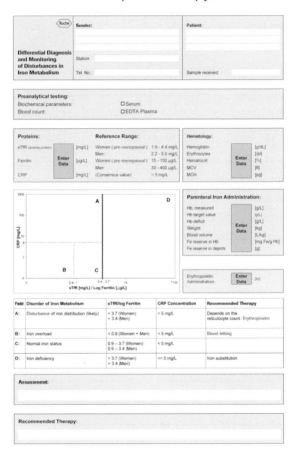

Fig. 28: Software program for performing successive diagnostics in cases of suspected disturbances of iron metabolism [183]

Most Frequent Disturbances of Iron Metabolism and Erythropoiesis

Erythropoietin (EPO) is the most important growth factor for regulating erythropoiesis. As shown in Figure 29, the regulation of erythropoiesis is controlled primarily by iron in addition to the growth factor EPO.

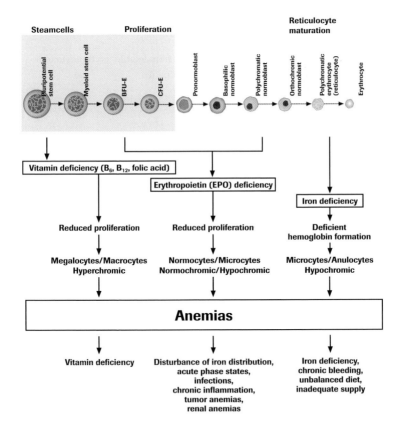

Fig. 29: Disturbances of erythropoiesis caused by deficiencies of vitamins, growth factors (EPO) and iron. Schematic illustration according to Thomas L. (2001) [184]

Clinical Aspects

Hypochromic, Microcytic Anemias

The most frequently-occurring iron metabolism anemias are iron deficiency and disturbances of iron distribution. They are hypochromic anemias and are often microcytic or normocytic. Medical practices currently dedicate significant resources to clarifying these types of anemia. In addition to iron deficiency, which is widespread, disturbances of iron distribution caused by tumors, infections or chronic inflammations are increasing markedly. A very clear classification of anemias has been used in hematological diagnostics for years (Tab. 15).

Table 15: Classification of anemias based on hemoglobin, erythrocyte indices (MCH, MCV) and reticulocyte count

	microcytic	normocytic	macrocytic
Hb (g/dL)	M < 13.5 W < 12.5 Ch < 11.5	M 14 – 17.5 W 12.5 – 15.5 Ch 11.5 – 15.5	M >18 W > 16 Ch > 16
MCH (pg)	hypochromic < 28 pg/cell	normochromic 28 – 33 pg/cell	hyperchromic > 33 pg/cell
MCV (fl)	microcytic < 80	normocytic 80 – 96	macrocytic > 96
Reticulocyte count (‰ of erythrocyte count)	hyporegenerative < 5	normoregenerative 5 – 15	hyperregenerative > 15

M = Men, W = Women, Ch = Children

In addition to the hemoglobin value, the erythrocyte indices

MCH = Hemoglobin content of erythrocytes or the mean cellular hemoglobin
MCV = Mean cell volume of erythrocytes

are the most important analytes that are automatically determined by all modern cell instruments. Their determination is indispensable to the clarification of hypochromic anemias (Fig. 30).

Clinical Aspects

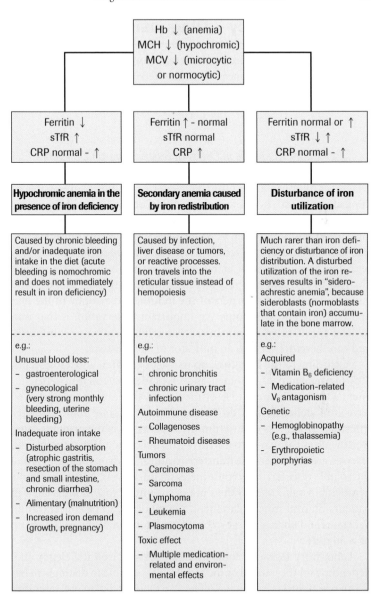

Fig. 30: Diagnosis of hypochromic anemias

Clinical Aspects

Iron Deficiency – Diagnosis and Therapy

In the case of a negative iron balance, the iron stores are reduced first; this can be seen from the measurement of ferritin. The concentration of active iron decreases only at a relatively late stage (as shown by the lower transferrin saturation or the higher transferrin receptor concentration).

Laboratory Diagnosis in Cases of Suspected Iron Deficiency

Diagnosis of non-manifest iron deficiency is practically impossible by clinical methods. The subjective condition of patients with iron deficiency does not reveal any definitely attributable changes. The familiar clinical symptoms such as pallor, weakness, loss of concentration, exertional dyspnea, and reduced resistance to infection appear only with the development of active iron anemia. The relatively specific changes in the skin and mucous membranes, atrophic glossitis and gastritis, cracks at the corners of the mouth, and atrophy of the hair and nails are late symptoms. An important observation is that iron deficiency very often accompanies serious, life-threatening conditions, and can therefore serve as an indicator of such diseases.

According to the literature, up to 5% of children and adolescents, 10% of premenopausal women, and 1% of men have an iron deficiency anemia. Approximately 15% of men and women over the age of 60 have iron deficiency, as do 25 to 40% of nursing home patients. Intestinal blood loss due to tumors or parasites is the primary cause worldwide as compared to nutritive iron deficiency. If the storage iron reserves are exhausted, the transferrin saturation drops below 15% and the soluble transferrin receptor increases intensively. A decrease in the hemoglobin value usually does not occur until 1 to 2 months later. In patients on oral iron replacement, the increased sTfR concentration decreases and normalizes at < 5 mg/L with ferritin values in the serum of > 30 µg/L.

Laboratory tests can confirm a diagnosis of iron deficiency and, depending on the pattern of the results, it is possible to distinguish between prelatent, latent, and manifest iron deficiencies. In prelatent iron deficiency, the body's iron reserves are reduced. Latent iron deficiency is characterized by a reduced supply of iron for erythropoiesis. This gives way to manifest iron deficiency, which is characterized by typical iron deficiency anemia.

Prelatent iron deficiency, which is equivalent to storage iron deficiency, is characterized by a negative iron balance. The body's reaction is to increase the intestinal absorption or iron. Histochemically, the iron content of bone marrow and of liver tissue decreases. The concentration of the iron transport protein transferrin in the blood increases as a measure of the increased intestinal absorption.

The consumption of storage iron is most easily detected by quantitative determination of the ferritin concentration, which typically falls to less than 20 ng/ml. The ferritin that can be detected in the circulating blood is directly related to the iron stores, and can thus be used as an indicator. The determination of ferritin has almost entirely replaced the determination of iron in bone marrow for the assessment of stocks of reserve iron. The determination of the soluble transferrin receptor (sTfR) is becoming increasingly important in the assessment of the erythropoietic activity [148].

With consumption of reserve iron, or when the iron stores are completely empty, the replenishment of iron for erythropoiesis becomes negative. The total loss of storage iron is indicated by a decrease in the ferritin concentration to less than 12 mg/L. An indication of the inadequate supply of iron for erythropoiesis is a decrease in the transferrin saturation to less than 15%; the sTfR values are above the normal range of > 5 mg/L. As a morphological criterion, the number of sideroblasts in the marrow falls to less than 10%. There are no noticeable changes in the red blood count at this stage of latent iron deficiency.

The laboratory results in this stage are characterized by a fall in the ferritin concentration in the blood to less than 12 mg/L and a fall in the hemoglobin concentration to less than 12 g/dl. A morphological effect of manifest iron deficiency is that the erythrocytes become increasingly hypochromic and microcytic. The mean cell volume (MCV) decreases to less than 80 fl, the mean cellular hemoglobin (MCH) is less than 28 pg and the mean cellular hemoglobin concentration (MCHC) may fall to less than 33 g/dl. The erythrocytes in the peripheral blood count are smaller than normal, and pale in the center. These altered erythrocytes are known as anulocytes. The morphological change in the blood count does not appear immediately, but only after the normochromic erythrocyte population has been replaced by the hypochromic microcytic erythrocytes in the course of the natural process of renewal. Iron deficiency is by no means ruled out by normochromic normocytic anemia. Pronounced hypochromia and microcythemia indicate that the iron deficiency has already been in existence for at least several months (Fig. 31).

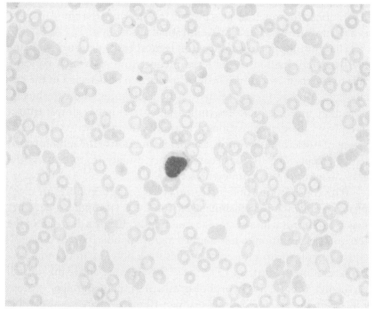

Fig. 31: Anulocytes

A hypochromic microcytic anemia is not necessarily an iron deficiency anemia. However, a morphologically characterized anemia accompanied by a ferritin value of less than 12 mg/L can always be identified as an iron deficiency anemia, and there is then, for the present, no need for further tests (Fig. 32).

It is extremely important in differential diagnosis to distinguish between the common iron deficiency anemias and other hypochromic anemias, since this has considerable implications for therapy. Only iron deficiency anemia responds to iron replacement. For patients suffering from other hypochromic anemias, the unnecessary administration of iron would lead to a risk of iron overload.

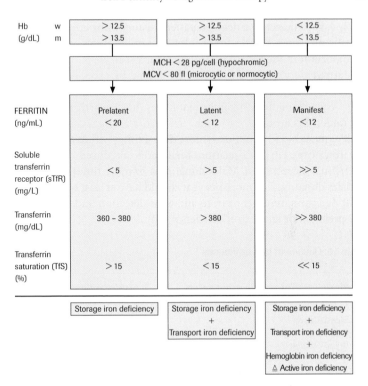

Hb w (g/dL) m	> 12.5 > 13.5	> 12.5 > 13.5	< 12.5 < 13.5
	MCH < 28 pg/cell (hypochromic) MCV < 80 fl (microcytic or normocytic)		
FERRITIN (ng/mL)	Prelatent < 20	Latent < 12	Manifest < 12
Soluble transferrin receptor (sTfR) (mg/L)	< 5	> 5	>> 5
Transferrin (mg/dL)	360 – 380	> 380	>> 380
Transferrin saturation (TfS) (%)	> 15	< 15	<< 15
	Storage iron deficiency	Storage iron deficiency + Transport iron deficiency	Storage iron deficiency + Transport iron deficiency + Hemoglobin iron deficiency △ Active iron deficiency

Fig. 32: Laboratory findings in the presence of iron deficiency

Clinical Pictures of Iron Deficiency

Iron deficiency occurs as a sign of increased physiological iron requirements during growth, as a result of menstruation, in pregnancy, and
during breast-feeding. The main cause of pathological iron deficiency,
on the other hand, is loss of blood, usually from the gastrointestinal
tract, though also from the urogenital tract in the case of women, and
less commonly in both sexes as a result of renal and bladder hemor-
rhages. Iron deficiency can also be caused by disturbed absorption of
iron (malabsorption), in which case it is important to check for any
medication that interferes with the absorption of iron. The clinical pictures of latent or manifest iron deficiency following blood loss are rela-

tively easy to detect by a detailed patient history or by appropriate diagnostic measures. Checks for occult blood in the stools are particularly important in the case of gastrointestinal losses.

Iatrogenic iron deficiency may be caused by excessive laboratory tests or by drugs, such as non-steroidal antirheumatic drugs or antacids. Asymptomatic gastrointestinal losses due to corticosteroids also fall under this heading.

Frequent blood donations (more than 4 times within a year) empty the iron stores. Further donations then lead to a reduced - but constant - ferritin concentration. Males donating 4 or more times per year and females donating 2 or more per year should have at least one ferritin or sTfR determination per year, to allow for detection and treatment of any prelatent or latent iron deficiency [90].

Table 16: Causes of iron deficiency

1. Physiological increase in requirements	3. Malabsorption
• Growth phase	• Sprue
• Menstruation	• Gastric resections
• Pregnancy	• Chronic atrophic gastritis
• Breast-feeding	• Drugs
2. Blood loss	**4. Inadequate supply**
• Gastrointestinal	• Unbalanced diet
– Esophagus	• Old age
– Varices	• New vegetarians
– Ulcers	
– Tumors	
– Inflammations	
– Malformation (blood vessels)	
• Urogenital	
– Hypermenorrhea	
– Birth	
– Tumors of the urinary tract	
– Calculi	
• Iatrogenic	
– Laboratory testing (excessive)	
– Drugs	
– Blood donors	

Clinical Aspects

Disturbances of iron absorption are known to occur after gastric resections (often associated with vitamin B_{12} deficiency) and in chronic atrophic gastritis. Malabsorption may also be induced iatrogenically by long-term tetracycline therapy, such as is often used for the treatment of acne. Idiopathic sprue generally also leads to iron malabsorption and hence to anemia.

Special consideration must also be given to certain population groups in which iron deficiency is common; these include infants and adolescents, the elderly, competitive athletes, and individuals having an unbalanced diet.

Behavioral disturbances in children can often be traced to latent or manifest iron deficiency. Intellectual and especially cognitive development in childhood is also adversely affected by iron deficiency. The observed symptoms can be eliminated by oral administration of iron. There is some debate as to whether brain development is permanently damaged by iron deficiency in early childhood. Iron deficiency in adolescence, especially in girls, is aggravated by poor eating habits. The supply of iron often corresponds to only 50% of the recommended amount, and this, coupled with puberty, leads to iron deficiency.

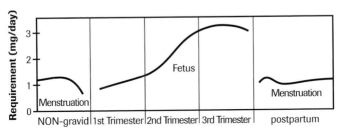

Fig. 33: Iron requirement during pregnancy

Latent iron deficiency is found in more than 50% of all pregnant women. The physiological course of pregnancy explains why latent iron deficiency appears mainly in the final three months. The ferritin concentration is a reliable parameter for the detection of iron depletion and deficiency in this situation. The daily iron requirement increases to 5-6 mg during the last three months of pregnancy, and this amount cannot be absorbed even from the best possible diet. Oral iron replacement is therefore necessary (Fig. 33).

Iron deficiency in the elderly, particularly those who live alone or in an institution, appears to be caused mainly by diet [164].

Special note should be given to iron deficiency in athletes of both sexes who take part in endurance sports. Iron deficiency in runners is mainly due to gastro-intestinal losses after long-distance running. Latent iron deficiency has also been found in long-distance swimmers. In endurance sports, a hemolytic influence apparently is an additional factor [159].

Extremely unbalanced diets have recently attracted considerable numbers of adherents. Iron deficiency anemia develops here mainly if the diet has an extremely high content of indigestible roughage [22].

Therapy of Iron Deficiency

Iron is one of the most important biocatalysts. As a central element of hemoglobin, it is essential to life. It can be administered orally as Fe(II) or in parenteral preparations as Fe(III).

Oral Administration of Iron

Oral replacement is always indicated in iron deficiency, which cannot be cured by taking in iron in the diet. In spite of various pharmaceutical formulations, the tolerability of oral iron preparations varies a great deal, so that each drug has to be monitored very carefully with regard to patient compliance.

When iron deficiency is present, the absorption of iron is up-regulated depending on the iron deficit. A bioavailability of 80 to 97% is achieved in the stomach and the proximal duodenum, but this requires that iron be supplied in an aqueous solution or released rapidly from the administered solution. If iron (ferroglycine sulfate) is administered in enteric-coated pellets, about 83% of it is absorbed. If the iron reserves are depleted, this portion can increase to 95% provided that iron is fully released [76]. A slow release of iron reduces absorption and, therefore, the bioavailability by about one-third, to approximately 60%. Iron(III) complexes administered orally are barely bioavailable and are therefore inefficient. The cause of the poor bioavailability lies in the fact that, in the case of iron(III) compounds, complete hydrolysis takes place at pH levels of just 2 to 4 and polymerization takes place in the small intestine at pH 7 to pH 8, forming insoluble and non-absorbable polynuclear iron(III)-hydroxide complexes which, due to their high molecular weight, cannot be absorbed. This reduces the bioavailability to less than 30%.

The bioavailability of oral iron preparations can be improved by ingesting it on an empty stomach, and this should be the rule. The simultaneous consumption of tea, coffee or dairy products in particular reduces the absorption of iron, as demonstrated in absorption studies with ferrous ascorbate solution. In the fasting state, about 10% was absorbed, although only about 1% was absorbed after breakfast. The extent of oral absorption is largely unrelated to the pharmaceutical formulation.

The gold standard of therapy is still iron sulfate, which is divided into 1 to 3 daily doses totalling 100 mg Fe(II). Taken on an empty stomach an iron absorption of 10-20 mg iron per day can be achieved [76]. A significant rise in the hematocrit can be expected within 3 weeks, and a normal red blood count (RBC) can generally be expected after 2 months if no further iron losses occur.

Iron therapy should be continued for a further 3-6 months after reaching a normal level in order to fill the body's iron stores. The ferritin level must be monitored during this period. Ferrous sulfate is suitable for oral administration of iron, as are ferrous sulfate, fumarate, chloride and lactate.

The most common iron compounds used for oral therapy are listed in Table 17. Fumarate and gluconate, in addition to iron sulfate, are commercially available in presentations ranging from tablets to coated tablets and suspensions. Of the absorption-enhancing substances, only

Clinical Aspects

Table 17: Recommended doses for the most common oral iron preparations

		Recommended dose
Ferrous sulfate	105 mg Fe^{2+}	Once daily
Ferrous fumarate	308 mg Fe-fumarate $\triangleq$ 100 mg Fe^{2+}	Once daily
Ferrous gluconate	200 mg Fe-gluconate $\triangleq$ approx. 30 mg Fe^{2+}	3 x 2 tablets daily
	625 mg Fe-gluconate/ascorbic acid $\triangleq$ 80 mg Fe^{2+}	1 – 2 tablets daily

ascorbic acid at a dosage of 200 mg or more has proved to be useful.

Oral iron preparations can cause gastrointestinal side-effects such as heartburn, nausea, flatulence, constipation and diarrhea. The intensity of the gastrointestinal side-effects depends on the dose and the speed at which the iron is released. Iron preparations with poor bioavailability, therefore, cause relatively few side-effects.

In order to avoid these difficulties it is advisable to start therapy with a small dosage and then gradually increase it. In approximately 25% of the patients, side-effects occur when a daily dosage of more than 100 mg iron is given, regardless of whether they are in the form of three equally divided doses or not. A rise in the side-effect rate to about 50% is observed in test persons when the orally administered iron dosage is doubled. The occurrence of heartburn or diarrhea is dependent on the administered dose.

As the oral absorption of iron in healthy persons is strictly regulated, it is virtually impossible to bring about symptoms of metal intoxication by excessive oral administration of iron to adults. Should this nevertheless occur, then hemochromatosis should be looked for. Fatalities in adults following oral administration of iron are generally the result of suicidal intent. The situation is different in children, particularly small children. A dose of just 1 or 2 g of iron can be fatal. Symptoms of iron intoxication can occur within 30 min but may also not develop until several hours have elapsed. They consist of cramp-like abdominal pain, diarrhea and vomiting of brown or bloody-stained gastric juice. The patients become pale or cyanotic, tired, confused, show incipient hyperventilation as a result of metabolic acidosis and die of cardiovascular failure.

In uncomplicated iron deficiency, hemoglobin or ferritin values increase 2 to 4 weeks after the start of iron therapy. STfR reaches a normal level within 2 weeks. The sTfR concentration usually normalizes when ferritin levels of 15 to 30 µg/L are reached.

In complicated iron deficiency (infection, inflammation, malignant tumor), an elevated sTfR concentration decreases as well after successful oral iron therapy. As the ferritin concentration can be normal or increases in the presence of tumor anemia or ACD despite inadequate iron supply for erythropoiesis, the drop in sTfR concentration alone is an indicator that an oral iron therapy is successful.

Parenteral Administration of Iron

The indications for i.v. iron administration are:

• poor iron absorption
• gastrointestinal disorders
• the inability to mobilize adequately large iron stores already present (renal insufficiency)
• intolerance of oral iron administration

Before administering iron parenterally, it is advisable to carry out an approximate calculation of the iron requirement and to administer it taking the iron reserves into account (Table 18).

Of the preparations available (iron saccharate, iron gluconate, iron ascorbate, iron citrate), iron saccharate has proved to be the most popular in Europe for parenteral administration. The iron saccharate complex has the advantage that it is not filtered through the glomeruli (molecular weight 43,000 D), is therefore not excreted renally and consequently cannot cause a tubulotoxic effect. Furthermore, the sub-

Table 18: Parenteral iron administration. Calculation of total dose required

Total amount of iron (g) = [Hb deficit x blood volume x iron reserve in Hb] + iron reserve in depots	
Example:	**Adult (male)**
BW (body weight)	70 kg
Blood volume:	0.069 l/kg x BW (body weight)
Hb (measured):	90 g/l blood
Hb (deficit):	40 g/l blood
Hb (target):	130 g/l
Iron reserve in Hb:	3.4 mg Fe/g Hb
Iron reserve in depots:	0.5 g (calculated by ferritin)*
Total iron dose required to increase the Hb value from 9 g/dL to 13 g/dL = [40 x 0.069 x 70 x 3.4 x 10^{-3}] + 0.5 = 0.7 + 0.5 = 1.2 (g)	

* 0.5 g iron reserves in the iron depots corresponds to a ferritin concentration of approx. 50 ng/mL. As a rule of thumb, 1 ng/mL ferritin equals approx. 10 mg iron in the iron stores.

Clinical Aspects

Table 19: Parenteral iron supplementation

Ferritin concentration	Iron saccharate	Iron gluconate
< 100 ng/mL Ferritin	40 mg Iron/HD*	62,5 mg Iron/HD*
> 100 ng/mL Ferritin	10 mg Iron/HD	10 mg Iron/HD

* Manufacturer's data for contents/bottle; HD hemodialysis

stance is characterized by its low potential for triggering an anaphylactic shock. However, it releases iron in the liver and from the complex and therefore hepatotoxicity should be watched for as a side-effect. When iron saccharate or iron gluconate are used, the iron doses per hemodialysis listed are acceptable according to the manufacturers' data.

The total dose for remedying a manifest iron deficiency anemia (ferritin < 12 ng/ml) is generally between 1 and 1.2 g iron administered parenterally.

Megaloblastic and macrocytic anemias as well as iron distribution disturbances, with or without iron deficiency, require somewhat more complex therapy.

Side-Effects and Hazards of Iron Therapy

Intravenous administration of iron is indicated above all in cases of functional iron deficiency.

During intravenous administration, intolerance reactions (immediately during or after intravenous administration) can occur. Undesired long-term side-effects in various systems of the body have also been described. Accordingly, intravenous iron therapy should only be carried out with strict adherence to the indications.

Immediate reactions include malaise, fever, acute generalized lymph adenopathy, joint pains, urticaria and occasionally exacerbation of symptoms in patients with rheumatoid arthritis.

These fairly harmless but unpleasant adverse reactions differ from the rare but feared anaphylactic reactions which can be fatal despite immediate therapy. Such reactions with fatal outcome have been reported occasionally particularly for iron dextran. These occurrences necessitate very strict indications for i.v. therapy [27]. There is confirmed evidence that infections, cardiovascular diseases and carcinogenesis can be influenced by the intravenous administration of iron.

There is a close relationship between the availability of iron and the virulence of bacterial infections. This can be explained by the fact that iron is a precondition for the multiplication of bacteria in the infected body. Excessive iron can therefore increase the risk of infection. It has already been shown in human and animal studies that the intravenous administration of iron during infection causes deterioration of the clinical picture. It has in the meantime been shown that hydroxyl radicals, which are formed during iron therapy, are responsible for the negative effects of iron. In other words, iron deficiency hinders bacterial growth but also hinders adequate defense against infection in the affected organism. Particularly in dialysis patients or patients with end-stage renal disease, intravenous iron therapy can negatively influence not only the activity of the phagocytes, but also that of the T- and B-lymphocytes [138].

In patients with malignoma, iron therapy is clearly indicated when iron deficiency exists. However, these patients frequently suffer from ACD in which it is known that functional iron is depressed even though the iron reserves are in the normal or elevated range. Administration of iron when not indicated cannot only have a detrimental effect on various organ systems of the sick person, but may also contribute to increased proliferation of neoplastic cells. Various studies have demonstrated that high transferrin saturation is associated with an elevated risk of carcinoma in general and of cancer of the lungs and colon in particular [118]. In a study comparing the relative cancer risk in blood donors and non-donors, there was a significant increase in the relative risk of non-donors for developing carcinoma [101].

A controversial point of discussion is the role that iron plays in the pathogenesis of cardiovascular disease and atherosclerosis. The hypothesis that iron depletion has a protective action against coronary heart disease was advanced as early as 1996 [174] to explain the striking difference between the sexes regarding the incidence of coronary heart disease. It is a fact that the virtual absence of myocardial infarction in women of child-bearing age is associated with low-depot iron levels. It is also striking that after cessation of the menstrual loss of iron there is a rapid rise in the number of cases of coronary heart disease [127].

The literature contains contradictory information about the relationship between iron pathogenesis and atherosclerosis: Ascherio has published a report stating that reduced levels of depot iron do not prevent the risk of coronary disease [7]. The same author reports that an increased dietary intake of hemoglobin iron in men leads to an increased risk of coronary disease even when cholesterol and fat intake are included in the risk assessment [8]. The importance of iron in atherosclerosis has been demonstrated by a number of studies. One of the most recent studies showed that serum ferritin values above 50 mg/L lead to a clear increase in atherosclerosis of the carotids in both men and women [100]. There are indications, however, that there is no association between serum ferritin, transferrin or dietary iron and the developmental stage of an atherosclerosis of the carotids [60].

Additionally, the NHANES II study ruled out high iron stores in an organism as the cause of cardiovascular disease and myocardial infarction [170].

The iron stores in the human body may influence physiological processes depending on age. Corti [39] demonstrated that the mortality risk and the risk of coronary heart disease increase with low iron levels in individuals over 70 years of age. An inverse correlation between serum iron levels and mortality risk apparently exists in this age group.

All observations that support the promotion of atherogenesis during intravenous iron therapy has led to considerations on the simultaneous use of erythropoietin and desferrioxamine in order to mobilize the iron depots and thus make intravenous administration of iron unnecessary. The difficulty associated with this therapy concept lies in the fact that the mobilization of depot iron cannot be predicted. A recently published study indicated that intravenous iron in combination with erythropoietin in dialysis patients increases the cardiovascular risk and, therefore, mortality [18].

In the light of the aspects discussed here, namely the influence of iron on infectious disease, carcinogenesis and the development of atherosclerosis, all indications are that stored iron is toxic. Every form of iron therapy therefore requires careful monitoring. The therapeutic goal is the achievement of normal values for hematocrit and hemoglobin.

Disturbances of Iron Distribution Diagnosis and Therapy

Chronic infections, tumors, chronic inflammations and autoimmune diseases "need" iron and withdraw it from hematopoiesis. "Secondary anemias", "anemias of infection or tumor anemias" or anemias of chronic disease (ACD) are the cause of a hypochromic anemia just as often as true iron deficiency. In addition to chronic inflammatory and neoplastic processes, they are observed primarily in patients with extensive tissue trauma. They are observed in the presence of chronic inflammatory and neoplastic processes as well as extensive tissue injuries.

Disturbances of Iron Distribution and Hypochromic Anemias

While the plasma ferritin concentration correlates with the body's total iron stores in patients with primary and secondary hemochromatoses, there are other conditions in which this correlation does not apply. Raised plasma ferritin concentrations are also found in patients with infection or toxin-induced damage to liver cells resulting from ferritin release in liver cell necroses, in patients with latent and manifest inflammations or infections, and in patients with rheumatoid arthritis. Raised plasma ferritin concentrations are also observed in patients suffering from physical and psychological stress, e.g. following serious trauma. In critically ill patients, plasma ferritin concentrations increase with increasing deterioration of the patient's clinical status, probably as a result of increased release from the macrophage system [20] - a non-representative raised plasma ferritin concentration exists (Tab. 20).

Table 20: Causes of iron displacement in patients with secondary anemias

Infections	• Chronic bronchitis
	• Chronic urinary tract infection
	• Chronic varicose complex or gangrene
	• Osteomyelitides
	• Tuberculosis
Tumors	• Carcinomas
	• Sarcoma
	• Lymphoma
	• Leukemia
	• Plasmacytoma
Autoimmune diseases	• Collagenoses
	• Rheumatoid diseases
Toxic effect	• Multiple drug- and environmentally-related effects

Clinical Aspects

The plasma ferritin concentration is not indicative of the body's total iron stores shortly after oral or parenteral iron therapy, or in patients with malignant tumors. As a basic rule, it can be assumed that a raised red blood cell sedimentation rate and/or pathological values for C-reactive protein (CRP) are likely to be accompanied by raised plasma ferritin concentrations.

The characteristics of these anemias are low serum iron concentrations combined with low transferrin saturation and an sTfR in the normal range. The iron storage protein ferritin is available in sufficient or elevated quantities. The morphology of the anemia is normocytic or microcytic.

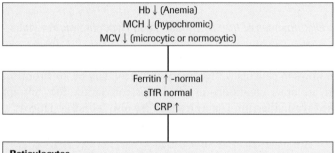

Hb ↓ (Anemia)
MCH ↓ (hypochromic)
MCV ↓ (microcytic or normocytic)

Ferritin ↑ -normal
sTfR normal
CRP ↑

Reticulocytes
- Almost always hyporegenerative in the presence of these secondary anemias (reticulocytes < 5 ‰).

The morphology of erythrocytes
- The erythrocytes are microcytic (MCV < 80 fl), of unusual shape and different sizes.

Inflammatory parameters
- CRP, red blood cell sedimentation rate (BSR), electrophoresis are changed, CRP is elevated in most cases.

Causes of secondary anemia in the presence of iron redistribution
are infections, liver diseases or tumors;
Iron travels into the reticular tissue instead of hematopoiesis

Fig. 34: Further laboratory findings in patients with secondary hypochromic anemias

Clinical Aspects

Iron and Cellular Immunity

The purpose of the immune system is to protect the organism from microorganisms, foreign substances, harmful substances, toxins and malignant cells. It makes use of the non-specific and the specific immune system.

The *non-specific immune system* consists primarily of the acid mantle of the skin, intact epidermis, intact complement system, antimicrobial enzyme systems and non-specific mediators such as interferons and interleukins. Granulocytes and monocytes/macrophages act at the cellular level.

The most important non-specific defense is the inflammatory reaction. As the first step in an inflammatory reaction, mediators (IL-1, IFN-γ) are released and increase the permeability of the capillary walls. Granulocytes and macrophages then enter the source of inflammation in order to phagocytize the causative agent.

The purpose of the *specific immune system* is to expand the antigen by cloning when inflammation occurs to enable a memory reaction in the future. T-lymphocytes formed in the thymus and B-lymphocytes formed in the bone marrow are specialized for this in particular. The maturation of T-lymphocytes takes place upon contact with dentritic cells and macrophages. This maturation process in the IL-12/IFN-γ cytokine environment results in CD4+ -THO cells and, finally, TH1 cells. The TH1 cells play a key role in the pathogenesis of disturbances of iron utilization in the presence of tumor anemias and anemias of infection and chronic inflammation (Fig. 35).

Dendritic cells (DC) are the most important cells of non-specific immunity in the body. T cells are able to stimulate immature DC to a limited extent; they are finally induced to mature into dentritic cells when affected by the inflammatory-acting cytokines TNF-α, IL-1, IL-6, LPS (lipopolysaccharide), bacteria and viruses.

Only terminally mature dendritic cells (DC) that were stimulated by CD40/CD40 ligands are able to produce large amounts of IL-12. This cytokine, in turn, induces the differentiation of CD4+ -THO cells in the direction of TH1 with release of interferon. Interferon-γ stimulates the antimicrobial and proinflammatory activity of macrophages and helps further the activation of cytotoxic T-cells (cytotoxic T-lymphocytes, CTL).

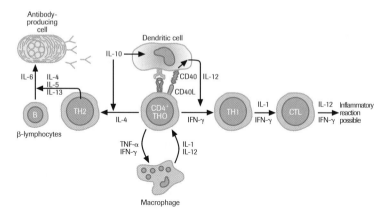

Fig. 35: Cell–cell interaction of cytokines in the differentiation of THO into TH1 and TH2 cells. According to Burmester G (1998) Taschenatlas der Immunologie: Grundlagen Labor, Klinik. Thieme, Stuttgart, New York and Moldawer et al [132]

Interleukins: IL-4, IL-5, IL-6, IL-10, IL-12, IL-13
IFN-γ = Interferon γ
CTL = cytotoxic T-lymphocytes
TH1, TH2 = Subpopulations of T-lymphocytes
CD40, CD40L = Cluster of differentiation (CD) 40 and 40L (according to the WHO-IUIS-
                    Standardization Committee of Leukocyte Differentiation Antigens)
B = β-lymphocyte
CD4+-T helper cell = CD44 is the antigen to the T helper cells
TNF-α = Tumor necrosis factor alpha

TH1 cells secrete interleukin-2, interferon-γ, TNF-β and GM-CSF and result, via macrophage activation, in pronounced inflammatory processes that enable the destruction of intracellular causative agents. The activation of macrophages results in the secretion of increased amounts of TNF-α. This reduces the production of antibodies and cell-destroying enzymes. Both of these induce an increase in TNF-α synthesis.

In the non-terminal differentiation of CD, e.g., when the T-cells do not express the CD40 ligands, or in the presence of IL-10, the differentiation of T-cells leans toward TH2, with the secretion of IL-4 and IL-5. Together with IL-13 and IL-6, these cytokines induce the maturation of B-cells in antibody-producing plasma cells, and the inflammatory cytotoxic T-cell response does not take place.

As illustrated in Fig. 35, the subpopulation of CD4+T helper cells (TH1) releases pro-inflammatory cytokines, which have a direct effect on iron metabolism, while the TH2 population is mainly responsible for the antibody response and does not directly affect iron metabolism.

The cytokines produced by TH1 subsets, such as interleukin-1 (IL-1) and tumor necrosis factor alpha (TNF-α), induce ferritin synthesis in cells of the non-specific immune system such as macrophages and hepatocytes, while interferon gamma (IFN-γ) withholds iron from the macrophages [193].

Increased release of cytokines such as IFN-γ and TNF-α, mediated by nitrogen oxide (NO), leads to an increased iron uptake in macrophages by an increased transferrin receptor expression. The increased iron uptake induces increased intracellular ferritin synthesis.

Iron intervenes in cellular immunity at many levels [196]. On the one hand, it affects the proliferation and differentiation of various lymphocyte subsets. On the other, it affects the immunopotential of macrophages [23, 24] by blocking the INF-γ-transmitted immune response in macrophages [194].

Iron-overloaded macrophages react more poorly to INF-γ, produce more TNF-α, and form more NO. The ceruloplasmin/haptoglobin system inhibits NO and directly affects the proliferation of the precursor cells of erythropoiesis. Additionally, the resistance to viruses and other intracellular pathogens is weakened. The withdrawal of metabolically active iron and its deposit as storage iron strengthens the organism's immune response to INF-stimulation [19, 130].

The regulatory antagonist of this stimulation mechanism lies in the reduction of the TH1-mediated immune reaction by IL-4 and IL-13. This is accomplished when these interleukins raise the intracellular concentration of iron by stimulating transferrin receptor expression. This is one of the basic mechanisms of the anti-inflammatory and macrophage-inhibiting effect [130].

Since iron is an important factor in the growth of tissue and microorganisms, iron deficiency limits DNA synthesis. Additionally, reduced hemoglobin synthesis and erythropoiesis is associated with a reduction in oxygen transport capacity, which causes a reduction in the supply of oxygen to rapidly growing tissues and microorganisms by the intracellular iron stores. Growth of noxae is inhibited as a result.

Clinical Aspects

Activation of the Immunological and Inflammatory Systems

Anemias due to chronic pathological processes (ACD) are the result of a multifactorial process in which activation of the immune and inflammatory systems play an important role.

Iron metabolism in monocytes/macrophages plays an especially significant role in chronic disease. The organism uses iron metabolism in the inflammatory and anti-neoplastic defense system. It draws iron from microorganisms and neoplastic cells and stores it in reticuloendothelial systems. This is characterized by the development of a normochromic or hypochromic, normocytic anemia. These types of anemia are caused by tumors, malignant growths, and chronic inflammations. Due to various cytokines, erythropoiesis is compromised primarily at the CFU-E level in this process.

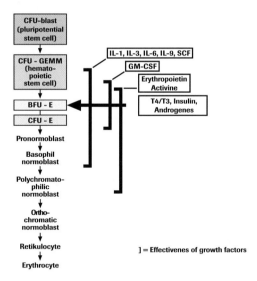

Fig. 36: **Differentiation of the hematopoietic system and regulation of the erythropoiesis by growth factors.**
CFU: colony forming unit; BFU: burst forming unit; E: erythrocytic; G: granulocytic; M: macrophagocytic; M: megaloblastic; IL: Interleukin; SCF: stem cell factor; GM-CSF: Granulocyte-macrophage colony-stimulating factor

Erythropoietin (EPO) is the most important and specific erythropoiesis-stimulating factor. It acts on early progenitor cells up to the maturation levels after the erythroblast. Without EPO, erythroid differentiation does not progress past the level of burst forming units (BFU-E).

Monocytes/macrophages play an important role in erythropoiesis in bone marrow. The progenitor cells of the red line proliferate and differentiate only under optimal local conditions. The blood islands in bone marrow consist of a centrally located macrophage surrounded by small cells of the erythroid and myeloid line. The surrounding cells also com-

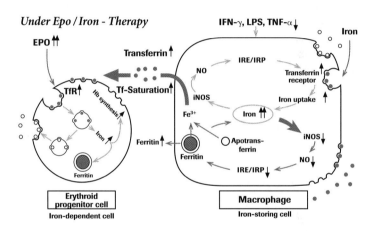

Fig. 37: Model of the autoregulatory loop between iron metabolism and the NO/NOS pathway in activated monocytes/macrophages and supply of an iron-dependent cell in a patient on EPO/iron therapy. Weiss G et al (1997) [195]

IFN-γ, interferon γ; iNOS = inducible nitric oxide synthase; IRE, iron-responsive element; IRE/IRP high-affinity binding of iron-regulatory protein (IRP) to IREs; LPS, lipopolysaccharide; TNF-α, tumor necrosis factor α; $\uparrow$ and $\downarrow$ indicate increase or decrease of cellular responses, respectively.

Supply of an iron-dependent cell.

Iron stored as ferritin within an iron-storing cell is released to transferrin, and then carried to the iron-requiring cell.

The cytoplasmic membrane of tissue cells contains transferrin receptors to which the iron-carrying transferrin binds.

The endosome migrates into the cytoplasm where it releases iron.

The endosome returns to the cytoplasmic membrane and apotransferrin is released into the extracellular space.

Explanation of signs: ⌣ transferrin receptor, ● iron-carrying transferrin,
                         ○ apotransferrin, ⊙ ferritin.

prise endothelial cells, fat cells, reticuloepithelial cells, and fibroblasts [196].

High concentrations of intracellular iron dramatically reduce the effect of IFN-γ on human monocytic cells. Iron regulates the cytokine effects in this process. Macrophages with high concentrations of intracellular iron lose the ability to phagocyt. After stimulation with IFN-γ and lipo-polysaccharides (LPS), cultivated macrophages produce increasing quantities of nitrogen oxide (NO), which is then converted to reactive nitrogen intermediates (RNI) such as nitrite and nitrate (Fig. 37).

An undesired effect in particular is the fact that availability of iron for hemoglobin synthesis is reduced. Iron replacement as part of erythro-poietin therapy stimulates erythropoiesis and iron uptake by the bone marrow cells on the one hand, and, on the other, withdraws iron from the macrophages and reduces the cytotoxic effects [197].

Iron and erythropoietin therapy can be assessed as very promising, since in addition to improving the anemia, the previously described inhibiting effect of iron on cytokine action and macrophage-induced cytotoxicity has a favorable influence.

With erythropoietin administration, the transferrin receptor on erythroid precursor cells is upregulated. A sequential administration of erythropoietin and iron (at intervals of 48 hours) should be discussed [193]. It is possible that negative reactions with regard to the immune response can be reduced [146].

Table 21: Biochemical background for EPO/Iron combination therapy

	Erythroid cells	Reticuloendothelial system (e. g. macrophages)
EPO ↑ = EPO treatment	• stimulates proliferation von of bone marrow erythroid cells • upregulates TfR expression	• upregulates transferrin receptor expression
„Free Iron" ↑ = i.v. iron treatment	• stimulates Hb synthesis	• inhibits NOS und NO production • upregulates ferritin expression • inhibits IFN-γ and TNF-α production

IFN-γ	=	Interferon-γ
TNF-α	=	Tumor necrosis factor α
NO	=	Nitric oxide
NOS	=	Nitric oxide synthesis

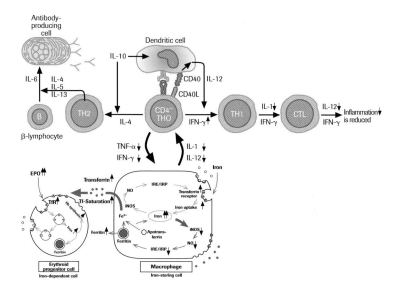

Fig. 38: Cytokines in the cell-cell interaction in the differentiation of T cells into TH1 and TH2 cells. T cells lead via macrophage activation to pronounced inflammatory processes. Via the cytokines there is a connection to the autoregulatory loop between iron metabolism in the macrophages and the NO/NOS pathway in activated macrophages. Metabolism is down-regulated with EPO and i.v. iron therapy. According to Moldawer et al. (1997) [132] and Weiss et al (1997) [195]

A combination of EPO/i.v. iron leads to a reduction of iron deposits in the macrophages and down-regulates the cytokine interaction and the inflammatory reaction, primarily of IL-1, IL-12 and IFN-g. The inflammatory activity is simultaneously inhibited. This explains the inflammation-inhibiting effect of EPO therapy and i.v. iron administration. When one considers that the therapy has no side-effects and that it not only leads to correction of anemia in patients with tumors and infections and in patients with chronic inflammation (e.g., rheumatoid arthritis), but to a correction in the inflammatory activity as well, it becomes clear that an important milestone in the therapy of these diseases has been reached.

Therapy with EPO and i.v. Iron Administration
– Down-Regulation of Inflammation

Recombinant human erythropoietin (rhEPO) produced using genetic engineering has been available for therapeutic use for various clinical pictures for about ten years. It was first tested in a clinical setting on dialysis patients who received regular blood transfusions to treat renal anemia. As chronic renal insufficiency progresses, the kidneys lose their ability to react to the drop in hematocrit by increasing synthesis adequately. The responsiveness of the bone marrow in patients on rhEPO is not impaired, however.

The clinical picture of renal anemia is a "classic" example for replacement therapy with rhEPO. Nor is it surprising that over 95% of

Table 22: Biological Function of EPO

Formation	• specialized kidney cells
	• Regenerating human liver cells
Regulation	• Hormones such as renin, angiotensin II or epinephrine
	• Cytokines such as IL-1, IL-6 or TNF
	• Oxygen supply at the site of EPO production
Biological function	• Growth factor with a hormone-like effect.
	• Precursor cells of the red blood cells (erythroblasts) in the bone marrow
	• Promotion of proliferation and differentiation of precursor cells in eythrocytes
EPO for disease	In patients with certain forms of anemia, especially aplastic renal anemia, the regulation of EPO formation in the kidneys appears to be intact. This leads to extremely high EPO concentrations in the serum of the individuals affected (up to 4 U/mL). Other forms of anemia, especially renal anemia, are characterized by serum EPO concentrations that are lower than expected for the severity of the anemia. The regulation of EPO formation is apparently disturbed in these individuals.
	Forms of anemia that may or may not be based on a deficit of erythropoietin. This question can be clarified by determining the erythropoietin concentration in serum and by relating the results to the hemoglobin concentration (or the hematocrit).
	Elevated values of erythropoietin accompanied by a normal or even raised hemoglobin concentration (and/or hematocrit values) were found in a number of diseases such as kidney and liver tumors or in patients with secondary forms of polycythemia. Polycythemia vera is characterized by an abnormally high number of red blood cells accompanied by a reduced serum titer of erythropoietin.

dialysis patients are successfully treated with rhEPO [86, 176].

Under physiological conditions, the neogenesis of erythropoietin takes place in the peritubular fibroblasts of the kidney. Under hypoxic conditions, synthesis of the hormone - mediated by a cellular oxygen sensor - increases (rise in the expression of the EPO gene). In patients with chronic renal insufficiency, these kidney cells lose their ability to adequately increase EPO formation.

There are a number of forms of anemia that are not due primarily to a deficit of EPO, but which can be corrected using rhEPO therapy. Almost all chronic inflammatory or malignant diseases are associated with an anemia. Many factors are significant with these anemias. First and foremost, the formation of red blood cells in the bone marrow is disturbed. Circulating cytokines released as part of the inflammatory process are responsible for causing the inhibition of erythropoiesis (TNF-α, IL-1, IL-6).

In patients with tumor anemias, anemias of infection, or anemias of chronic inflammatory diseases, the direct inhibition of erythropoiesis and the reduced formation of erythropoietin caused by the circulating cytokines, or the reduced release of iron from the reticuloendothelial system means that higher EPO doses are required to correct the anemia as compared to renal anemia. In many patients with carcinomas, infections or chronic intestinal disease or rheumatoid arthritis, however, the hematocrit can be increased, the need for transfusions can be reduced, and quality of life can be improved.

Anemias of Infection and Malignancy

The anemia of infections and malignancies, as well as anemia of chronic disease (ACD) are observed with greater frequency in internal medical practices than iron deficiency anemia. These anemias are caused by disturbances of iron distribution with insufficient recycling of iron from the storage iron compartment into the functional compartment. The erythropoietic precursor cells are supplied with inadequate amounts of iron even though the RES is filled with iron.

The hypoproliferation of erythropoiesis is induced by inflammatory cytokines (IL-1, IL-6, TNF-α). The erythropoiesis is adjusted for the reduced iron supply, so that normal hemoglobinization of the red blood cells takes place. This results in a normocytic, normochromic anemia with low erythrocyte count.

The clinical findings in patients with anemias of inflammation and malignancy are presented in Table 23. If these patients experience bleeding, however, a combination of iron deficiency and anemia of inflammation or malignancy may occur. Diagnosis of an active iron deficiency is difficult in such cases and cannot be clarified based on the laboratory parameters ferritin, transferrin saturation and soluble transferrin receptor (sTfR).

Table 23: Clinical findings in patients with anemia of infection, inflammation and malignancy, and clinical interpretation (Thomas et al.) [182, 183]

	Clinical findings	Clinical Interpretation
Hemoglobin	9 – 12 g/dL	Normochromic, normocytic anemia.
Erythrocytes	3 – 4 million/l	If accompanied by inadequate iron supply for
MCH	> 28 pg	erythropoiesis, hypochromic and microcytic
MCV	> 80 fl	erythrocytes are formed.
Reticulocytes-production index	< 2	Hypoproliferative erythropoiesis caused by a reduced erythropoietin effect.
Iron	< 40 µg/dL	Disturbance of iron distribution due to
Ferritin	> 100 µg/L	increasing storage in the macrophages of the
Transferrin	< 200 mg/dL	reticuloendothelial system.
Transferrin saturation	< 15 %	
sTfR normal		

MCH = Mean Cell Hemoglobin
MCV = Mean Cell Volume
sTfR = Soluble Transferrin Receptor

Biological Activity of Tumor Necrosis Factors (TNF)

Various cell types can produce TNF. Monocytes and macrophages are the main source of this cytokine. TNF induces a series of proinflammatory changes in endothelial cells as well as the production of additional proinflammatory cytokines, the expression of adhesion molecules, the release of procoagulatory substanced and the induction of iNOS (inducible nitric oxide synthase) [195].

The therapeutic success of blocking antibodies and receptor fusion proteins [161] underscores the importance of searching for further therapeutic strategies using this cytokine with the goal of effectively inhibiting TNF synthesis.

TNF–inhibiting substances:

- Substances that inhibit the formation of TNF, such as phosphodiesterase inhibitors, prostaglandins, adenosine, corticosteroids and interleukin 10.
- Substances that prevent the processing of the TNF-Pro protein by inhibiting the specific metalloproteinase.
- Substances that weaken the effect of the active TNF such as anti-TNF antibodies and TNF-receptor Fc fusion proteins.

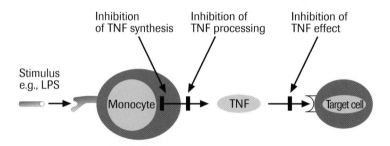

Fig. 39: The biological activities of the TNF. TNF are formed by monocytes / macrophages after stimulation with lipopolysaccharides (LPS). TNF can be inhibited at three levels: synthesis, processing, and the effect on target cells.
According to A. Eigler et al. (2001) Internist – 42: 28-34

Therapeutic Strategies for Malignancies

There are indications that the human body performs immune surveillance of tumors [165, 107]. Unlike bacteria and viruses, which are effectively detected and fought by the immune system, tumor cells often exhibit minimal changes in the protein pattern compared to normal cells. Individual peptides are usually the only potentially "foreign" antigens that can be detected and fought. Nevertheless, very successful antitumoral strategies have been developed in recent years in particular.

Strategies for treating tumors can be divided into two categories: therapeutic strategies directed toward the direct destruction of malignant tumor cells, and more recent approaches that aim to destroy tumor-supplying structures (tumor vessels and stroma) and thereby indirectly lead to the destruction of the tumor.

Ligands in the tumor necrosis factor family released in excess amounts appear to play a central role in the induction of malignant tumors [153, 192]. In addition to the classical low molecular-weight compounds, protein-based drugs have become important due to their highly-selective effect. Interest in these compounds is particularly high for the treatment of tumor diseases for which no therapeutic methods exist at this time. The molecular basis for the development of protein therapeutics are antibodies, cytokines and their receptors as well as recombinant derivatives and fusion proteins derived from these protein classes [190].

Early on in clinical investigations, attempts were made to use systematically applied TNF as an antitumor agent. These efforts were unsuccessful, however, as TNF elicits pronounced side-effects that can include induction of shock. The side-effects of a systemic TNF treatment are due primarily to its pleiotropic, proinflammatory effect and the ubiquitous distribution of TNF receptors. For this reason, ligands in the cytokine family of the tumor necrosis factor (TNF) have received the majority of attention recently.

A few very promising approaches are being pursued at this time using apoptosis-inducing molecules in the TNF family that have a strong cytotoxic effect on tumor cell lines [192]:

• Tumor targeting:
  The search for an antigen that is not tumor-specific. FAP (fibroblast activation protein), a molecule expressed on stromal fibroblasts of the stroma, is a membrane-bound protease that is a selective marker protein detectable in more than 90% of solid tumors [137]. As carcinoma typically comprise a high stroma portion, FAP is a universal and highly-expressed marker of solid tumors.

• Antibody-cytokine fusion proteins:
  Antibody-cytokine fusion proteins are being developed with the goal of improving antitumoral effectiveness while preventing systemic side-effects that limit therapy. FAP is chosen primarily as the target antigen for cytokines in the TNF family due to its dominant expres-

sion [153]. The goal in every case is to produce highly-effective deriva-tives -with no or reduced side-effects- of apoptosis-inducing ligands in the TNF family for tumor therapy. It cannot be foreseen at this time whether and which of the therapies for inhibiting the TNF will achieve clinical relevance. Reports of frequent occurrences of lym-phoma and carcinomas under therapy with anti-TNF antibodies are putting a damper on initial feelings of euphoria.

Hemoglobin Values in Therapies with Cytostatic Drugs

Randomized studies in patients with multiple myeloma (MM), non-Hodgkin's lymphoma (NHL) or chronic lymphatic leukemia (CLL) have made it clear that administration of EPO can raise hemoglobin and reduce a patient's need for transfusions [30, 115].

The hemoglobin value (Hb) is apparently an important factor in the quality of life in patients on virtually any cytostatic therapy. A large multi-centric, randomized study conducted by Littlewood et al. [115] inves-tigated the influence of EPO on the need for transfusions and the qual-ity of life of patients with solid tumors and hematological system diseases under chemotherapy that does not include cis-platinum. The study included patients with solid tumors or hematological neoplasias in which anemia (Hb < 10.5 g/dL) was diagnosed or in which the Hb value fell by more than 1.5 g/dL in the first four weeks of chemotherapy. The patients were treated with rhEPO (3 x 150 IU/kg/week) for 28 weeks in parallel with chemotherapy. Despite the chemotherapy, treatment with erythropoietin led to an increase in the hemoglobin value by 2 g/dL, in patients with solid tumors as well as patients with hematological neo-plasias.

Anemias in the presence of malignant tumors are therefore the result of a multifactorial process in which the immune system and the inflam-matory process play a dominant role [118, 119].

Known causes of anemias in patients with neoplasias are tumor-induced bleeding, hemolysis or infiltration of the bone marrow by tumor cells. The majority of anemias that occur in conjunction with malignant neoplasias are caused either directly or indirectly by the tumor itself, however. Anemia is the result of an imbalance between the rate of pro-duction of erythrocytes in the bone marrow and their dwell time in the blood. The tumor impairs the proliferation and life span of red blood cells. It is known that the life span of erythrocytes is shorted from 120 days to 60 – 90 days in patients with malignancies. The activation of the immune system in tumor-induced anemia apparently leads to a suppression of erythropoiesis, for which cytokines are responsible (TNF-α, IL-1, INF-γ).

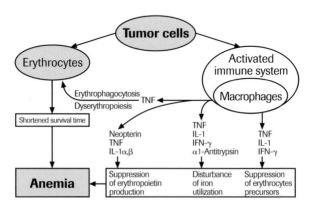

Fig. 40: Pathophysiological mechanisms in tumor-induced anemia.
          TNF = Tumor Necrosis Factor; IFN = Interferon; IL = Interleukin.
          Modified according to MR Nowrousian et al. (1996) [134]

The activation of erythropoiesis is regulated by the growth hormone erythropoietin, which is produced in the proximal tubuli of the kidney. In patients with tumor-induced anemias, exogenously supplied, recombinant erythropoietin stimulates the proliferation and well-differentiation of precursors of red blood cells. Erythropoietin and IFN-γ can be considered opponents in terms of their effect on erythropoiesis. IFN-γ inhibits the expression of the erythropoietin receptor. It is therefore understandable that recombinant erythropoietin counteracts the tumor-induced anemia.

The direct effect of interleukin 1 (IL-1), interferon gamma (IFN-γ) and tumor necrosis factor alpha (TNF-α) on bone marrow and erythropoietin production was detected in addition to the inadequate response to erythropoietin doses. The hemoglobin level above all is a prognostic factor. This was determined nearly 10 years ago in patients with small-cell lung carcinoma [119]. The participation of the bone marrow and the residual hematopoiesis - not the type of tumor - apparently are decisive factors in the success of therapy, as is the type, duration and intensity of chemotherapy. Chemotherapy schemes that contain platinol compounds exhibit a better reaction to erythropoietin doses. Interestingly enough, a low initial erythropoietin value, as one often finds primarily in patients with lymphoma and myeloma, is a good prognostic factor for a patient's response to therapy. An initial erythropoietin level of less than 250 IU/L is considered particularly favorable [117].

The prognosis of therapeutic success with solid tumors is more difficult, although a rise in the soluble transferrin receptor (sTfR) within two weeks after onset of therapy is considered a favorable prediction for therapeutic success. Ludwig et al. [118] report therapeutic successes in which an increase in hemoglobin concentration by more than 0.5 g/dL and a drop in the erythropoietin level to less than 100 IU/L was observed after 2 weeks. A drop in serum ferritin is also interpreted as a favorable sign for the therapy.

In the mean time, patients on radiotherapy have also been treated with erythropoietin. It was observed that the hemoglobin value increased among the patients with EPO, but it did not in the untreated control group.

Hypoxic regions exhibit increased resistance to radiation therapy. Apparently there is a correlation between the Hb value and the median oxygen partial pressure in the tumors. Since the hemoglobin concentration is the most important oxygen supply-determining parameter, an increase in the Hb value with EPO to over 12 g/dL in oncological patients appears reasonable, even if non-oncological patients typically are still capable of tolerating lower Hb values.

Erythropoietin and Iron Replacement in Tumor Anemias

Patients with malignant diseases often develop an anemia that is caused by the malignant process itself or the therapy. Various factors such as the type of tumor and the duration of illness, as well as the type and intensity of chemotherapy and/or radiotherapy influence the anemia rate.

Nearly 50 - 60% of patients who undergo aggressive chemotherapy to treat a malignant lymphoma, bronchial carcinoma, gynecological tumors or a carcinoma of the urogenital tract require blood transfusions. Blood transfusions are associated with numerous side-effects and risks, however (such as allergic reactions or infections such as hepatitis, HIV, bacterial contamination of the blood product or a blood group-incompatibility). An unavoidable side-effect of blood transfusions is chronic immune suppression. This is fatal in tumor patients in particular, as it can encourage tumor progression. Other side-effects include iron and volume overload.

These disadvantages can be prevented by administering recombinant human erythropoietin. EPO increases the Hb value in the physiological pathway and leads to improved quality of life in patients. EPO administration is therefore better tolerated and has a favorable influence on the results of cancer treatment. Tumor hypoxia and anemia are negative prognostic indicators in terms of the results of treatment of solid and hematological carcinomas [119].

The treatment of anemia while simultaneously reducing transfusions is already being used, in addition to chemotherapy treatment, very successfully in patients
• with solid tumors
• with malignant lymphomas (e.g., chronic lymphatic leukemia [CLL], Hodgkin's lymphoma [HL], non-Hodgkin's lymphoma [NHL])
• with multiple myeloma (MM)
• who have an increased transfusion risk due to their general condition (e.g., cardiovascular status, anemia)
• on chemotherapy with platinum-derivatives and chemotherapy drugs that do not contain platinum.

As a result of a patient's response to therapy with erythropoietin, the need for erythrocyte concentrate transfusions drops substantially. In a clinical study conducted by Leon et al. [108] to analyze the erythrocyte requirement under chemotherapy, only 16% of patients treated with erythropoietin required a transfusion. The same observation was described by Qvist et al. [149].

Clinical experience shows that the following response rates are obtained under a dosage of erythropoietin of 150 IU/kg body weight (approx. 10 000 IU), 3 times a week:

Table 24: Response rates in patients with malignant diseases to recombinant human erythropoietin and the portion of patients with endogenous erythropoietin deficiency

Clinical picture recombinant	Endogenous erythropoietin deficiency [%]	Response rates to erythropoietin [%]
NHL	38	50 – 61
CLL	53	approximately 50
CMS	59	variable
MM	80	50 – 80
MDS	-	8 – 28
Solid tumors	86	40 – 62
After chemotherapy	50 – 80	52 - 82

NHL	Non-Hodgkin's lymphoma
CLL	Chronic Lymphatic Leukemia = Chronic Lymphatic Lymphoma
CMS	CMS Chronic Myeloic Leukemia = Chronic Myeloproliferative Syndrome
MM	Multiple Myeloma, MDS Myelodysplastic Syndrome

According to this information, more than half of the patients with NHL, CLL or MM respond very well to erythropoietin. Good to very good response rates are typically found in patients with solid tumors and with chemotherapy-induced anemias as well.

The response rates in patients with myelodysplastic syndrome (MDS), in contrast, is low, i.e., less than 10%. This is likely due to the fact that a disturbance of iron utilization exists here [119]. Investigations conducted by Mantovani [124] indicate that erythropoietin does not affect the immunological parameters IL-1, IL-6 or TNF-α in these tumor patients.

The following indications for treatment with erythropoietin in patients with malignancies are clinically promising (Tab. 25):

Table 25: Indications with EPO treatment of malignancies

- Prevention of iatrogenic hemosiderosis and transfusion reactions

- Multiple myeloma (MM) when serum erythropoietin is below 100 IU/L

- Non-Hodgkin's lymphoma (NHL), Hodkin's disease with bone marrow infiltration and therapy with monoclonal antibodies

- Myelodysplastic syndrome (MDS) when serum erythropoietin is below 100 IU/L

- Chronic myeloproliferative syndrome (CMS), depending on the extent of bone marrow insufficiency

Clinical Aspects

The most important predictive parameter for response to EPO therapy is functional iron deficiency (ferritin value > 20 µg/L, soluble transferrin receptor (sTfR) > 5 mg/L). Functional iron deficiency is one of the most important factors that influence the response to EPO. Intravenous iron administration is therapeutically efficient. Elimination of the functional iron deficiency is best accomplished by parenteral iron substitution with a ferrous saccharate complex.

Further important predictors at the onset of therapy are the endogenous EPO serum level and the thrombocyte count. Low serum erythropoietin values at the onset of therapy (< 250 IU/L) and normal thrombocyte counts (> 100 x 109/L) are therefore independent prognostic factors that indicate a response.

Beginning in week 2 to 4, relative changes in reticulocytes, the Hb value, and the transferrin receptors in the serum represent good starting points. The prediction as to whether the patient will respond to EPO or not makes it possible to achieve maximum effectiveness and, therefore, to minimize costs.

In addition to rh-EPO, recombinant DNA technology has made it possible to synthesize an analog to rh-EPO, Novel Erythropoiesis Stimulating Protein (NESP) [51,120], which makes longer administration intervals possible [51], as its half-life is three times as long as that of rHu-EPO. 200 IU rHu-EPO is roughly equivalent to 1 µg NESP [66]. Antibodies to NESP have yet to be detected in the serum of treated patients [65].

The therapy of anemias of infections, tumors and chronic inflammation is characterized by inadequate erythropoietin secretion and can be effectively corrected by the use of rHu-EPO or NESP when the functional iron deficiency was eliminated previously in timely fashion by iron doses.

The recommended erythropoietin dose is approximately 150 IU rHu-EPO/kg body weight three times a week. This corresponds to about 450 IU rHu-EPO/kg body weight once a week. For 70 kg/body weight, this works out to about 31,000 IU rHu-EPO or 15 µg NESP.

Recent investigations have shown that the administration of 150 U/kg body weight of erythropoietin i.v. three times a week can be replaced with a dose of approximately 30,000 IU subcutaneously once a week beginning with chemotherapy.

Hemoglobin increases in the target range under this therapeutic regimen as well, and the transfusion requirement drops dramatically. In a study conducted by Cheung [33], the clinical effect as well as similar pharmacodynamics were observed with equally good clinical results. The same observations were reported in a study by Gabrilove [61], in which patients reported a distinct improvement in quality of life, which was significantly related to the rise in hemoglobin concentration.

In the present studies, the one-time high-dosage administration of erythropoietin shows the same results as the dose three times a week, but it clearly has the advantage that patient care is more pleasant. It is likely that the intervals of the once-per-week administration of NESP can be extended.

Table 26: Combined dose of EPO/i.v. iron in the treatment of tumor anemias

EPO	IU/week	approx. 30 000
i.v. iron	mg/week	< 20
Target Hb	g/dL	12
Target ferritin	µg/L	100 – 300
Target soluble transferrin receptor (sTfR)	mg/L	< 5
Target transferrin saturation (TfS)	%	> 15
Target CRP	mg/L	< 5

ACD	=	Anemia of chronic disease
TfS	=	Transferrin saturation
sTfR	=	Soluble transferrin receptor
Hb	=	Hemoglobin
CRP	=	C-reactives protein

In order to best care for patients who receive rHu-EPO in combination with i.v. Fe(III) injections, the essential diagnostic parameters of iron metabolism should be determined at regular intervals during treatment (Tab. 27).

Clinical Aspects

Table 27: Diagnostic parameters and expected values for iron replacement under EPO therapy in patients with tumor anemia

Diagnostic parameter	Expected values	Frequency of determination
Hemoglobin	12 g/dL	
Hematocrit	30-36 %	quarterly
Reticulocytes	10-15 ‰	
Folate	> 20 ng/mL	semi-annually
Vitamin B_{12}	> 2 ng/mL	
Ferritin	100-300 ng/mL	
Soluble transferrin receptor (sTfR)	< 5 mg/L	
Transferrin saturation	20-30 %	At the beginning and then quarterly
Hypochromic erythrocytes	< 10 %	
CRP	< 5mg/L	

All hematological parameters and iron parameters should be determined at the onset of therapy with rHu-EPO and with i.v. iron. These parameters should be tested twice a year.

Anemias of Chronic Inflammatory Processes

The cellular immune system (granulocytes, monocytes/macrophages, natural killer cells, T- and B-lymphocytes) is involved in all inflammatory processes and especially in chronic inflammations such as infections, malignant growth, skeletal diseases such as rhematoid arthritis, collagenoses and autoimmune diseases.

After the discovery of the proinflammatory proteins interleukin-1 (IL-1) and tumor necrosis factor alpha (TNF-α) and their role in septic shock, substances were developed to quickly neutralize them. At the same time, the relationships between disease activity of rheumatoid arthritis (RA) and IL-1 and TNF-α were becoming better understood [161]. Technological advances in the production of humanized monoclonal antibodies and initial good experiences in the therapy of RA with anti-CD4 antibodies paved the way for long-term treatment of rheumatoid arthritis (RA) and other chronic inflammatory diseases with IL-1/TNF-α binding substances [122].

Anemias of Rheumatoid Arthritis (RA)

Due to a chronic inflammatory process, rheumatoid arthritis leads to the gradual, progressive destruction of joint cartilage and bone. The disease is not limited to joints, however. It is also frequently manifested in other organs such as the heart, eyes, and kidneys.

In every case, the joints become inflamed. This inflammation is accompanied by a strong, painful swelling of the synovial membrane. Connective tissue then proliferates in the cartilage, which eventually destroys the joint cartilage and the exposed bone. In cases of pronounced activity, the patient also suffers from anemia and thrombocytosis (Fig. 41).

Neutrophils accumulate in the synovial fluid, while macrophages and T-lymphocytes in particular accumulate in the synovial membrane. Cell infiltration and the regeneration of blood vessels cause the synovial membrane to thicken (formation of pannus). During this process, large quantities of macrophages are located in the border of the synovial membrane and in the cartilage contact zone. The macrophages and fibroblasts are induced via proinflammatory cytokines (e.g., TNF-α, IL-1) to release collagenase and stromelysin 1, two matrix metalloproteinases that play a significant role in the destruction of cartilage. Osteoclasts are stimulated (Fig. 41).

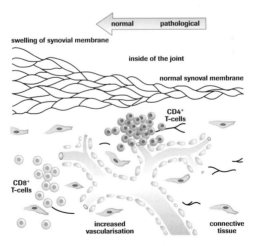

Fig. 41: Cell structure of the synovialis

Cytokine-Induction

Excess quantities of released tumor necrosis factor alpha (TNF-α) - which are secreted by activated monocytes, macrophages and dentritic cells, and IL-1, the main task of which is macrophage activation - play a central role in the induction of rheumatoid arthritis. Both cytokines suppress via activation of interferon (IFN) the formation of CFU-E (colony forming unit - erythrocytic) and, depending on their concentration, they intervene massively in the erythropoietic maturation sequence and the biological activity of erythropoietin. TNF-α and IL-1 (via INF-γ) are antagonists of EPO. High concentrations of TNF-α and IL-1, due to the massive destruction of erythropoiesis, can lead to hypochromic anemia (Fig. 42).

Table 28: Laboratory diagnostics of rheumatoid diseases

	CRP	Rheumatoid factor	ASL, ADNASE	ANA
Rheumatoid arthritis	++	++	-	+
Rheumatic. fever	+	(+)	++	(+)
Collegenoses e. g., SLE	(+)	(+)	-	+++

CRP   = C-reactive protein
ASL   = antistreptolysin titer
ADNASE = streptodornase
ANA   = antinuclear antibodies
SLE   = systemic lupus erythematodes

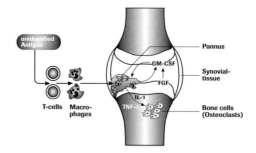

Fig. 42: Induction of rheumatoid arthritis. (According to Burmester G (1998)
         Taschenatlas der Immunologie: Grundlagen Labor Klinik.
         Thieme, Stuttgart, New York).
         FGF = Fibroblast growth factor; GM-CSF = Granulocyte macro-
         phage/monocyte colony-stimulating factor

Therapeutic Strategies of Rheumatoid Arthritis

The use of anti-inflammatory substances such as non-steroidal anti-rheumatics, glucocorticoids, antimetabolites (methotrexate), and immunosuppressants has been established for years to treat chronic polyarthritis.

The therapeutic possibilities for treating RA effectively and sustainably have often been inadequate. This has prompted increased efforts in recent years to develop and clinically evaluate immunobiological substances ("biological" therapeutics). Special attention is being given to proinflammatory cytokines and special TNF-α as a target molecule for developing new effective therapeutic principles. Two biological TNF-α-blocking substances for treating patients with RA are available at this time [161]:

• The chimeric TNF-α-neutralizing monoclonal antibody CA-2 (Infliximab) and

• the soluble TNF-α receptor p75 IgG1 fusion construct (Etanercept)

The long-term effects of both therapeutic possibilities cannot yet be assessed, although lymphoma neogenesis must be feared from both [Fig. 42].

A further biologically active substance that will be available shortly is a recombinant interleukin-1 receptor antagonist (IL-1Ra).

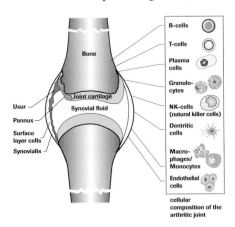

Fig. 43: Cells in the arthritic joint. According to Burmester G (1998) Taschenatlas der Immunologie: Grundlagen Labor, Klinik. Thieme, Stuttgart, New York

[1] Generic name for Anti-TNF monoclonal antibody, cA2, CenTNF, TA650
[2] Generic name for soluble tumor necrosis factor receptor, TNF receptor fusion protein

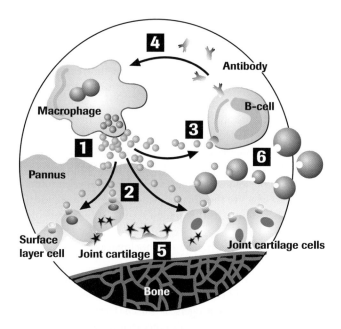

Fig. 44: Blockage of inflammation courses in the joints: 1. Macrophages in the synovial fluid excrete TNF-α . 2. TNF releases collagenases and other metaloproteinases that play a significant role in the destruction of cartilage. Cell infiltration causes the synovial membrane to thicken (formation of Pannus). 3. TNF stimulates B-cells to produce antibodies. 4. The antibodies initiate in the macrophages the synthesis of additional TNF. 5. The metalo-proteinases attack the synovial cells, the joint cartilage and destroy bone cells. 6. Tumor necrosis factor-(TNF-) blocking antibodies neutralize raised levels of TNF.

Erythropoietin and Iron Therapy of Rheumatoid Arthritis (RA)

Iron metabolism in monocytes/macrophages plays an especially significant role in chronic disease. The organism uses iron metabolism in the inflammatory and anti-neoplastic defense system. It draws iron from microorganisms and neoplastic cells and stores it in reticuloendothelial systems. This is characterized by the development of normochromic, normocytic anemia (ACD = Anemias of Chronic Disease). This type of anemia is caused by all types of inflammation (rheumatoid arthritis, malignant growths, or trauma). Due to various cytokines (TNF-α, IL-1, IL-6, INF-γ), erythropoiesis is compromised primarily at the CFU-E level in this process.

Iron and erythropoietin therapy in patients with chronic inflammation can be assessed as promising [32, 133], as in addition to improving the anemia, the previously described inhibiting effect of iron on cytokine action and macrophage-induced cytotoxicity has a favorable influence.

As under erythropoietin administration the transferrin receptor on erythroid precursor cells is upregulated. The sequential administration of erythropoietin and iron (at intervals of 48 hours) should be discussed [193, 195].

Initial therapeutic results are very encouraging [99]. Concomitant anemia, which is severe in some cases, can be successfully treated by erythropoietin substitution [98]. The patients were treated with 150 IU rhEPO per kg body weight twice weekly over a period of 12 weeks. Where there was a functional iron deficit, the patients were additionally given 200 mg Fe^{3+}-sucrose weekly i.v.

All patients showed normalization of Hb concentration and quality of life as measured by various parameters such as multi-dimensional assessment of fatigue (MAF) and muscle strength index (MSI). Laboratory parameters for the activity of rheumatoid arthritis and rheumatoid arthritis disease activity index (RADAI) also showed a clear improvement during erythropoietin therapy. Upon cessation of therapy after the 12-week period there was - as expected - a decrease in the improvement achieved.

In order to achieve optimum management of patients treated with rhEPO in combination with intravenous iron injections, the iron balance parameters listed in Table 29 should be determined at regular intervals. Recommendations for the treatment of anemia in RA have been updated. At the moment, virtually identical recommendations apply both to the treatment of anemia in RA (iron distribution disorder) and to anemia due to renal failure (erythropoietin deficiency and iron utilization disorder) (Table 29). Treating patients with rhEPO has proven over many years to be very reliable therapy, in particular due to the absence of side-effects.

Clinical Aspects

Table 29: Combined administration of EPO/i.v. iron in the treatment of ACD

Correction			Monitoring		
EPO	IU/kg/week	3 x 50 – 150	3 x 50 – 150	IU/kg/week	
i.v. iron	mg/week	10 – 40	i.v. iron	mg/week	10 - 20
Target Hb	g/dL	12	Hb	g/dL	12
Target Ferritin	µg/L	100 – 300	Ferritin	µg/L	100 – 300
Target s-Trans-ferrin-Receptor (sTfR)	mg/L	< 5	sTfR	mg/L	< 5
Target transferrin-saturation (TfS)	%	> 15	Transferrin-saturation (TfS will be replaced by TfR in future)	%	> 15 – 45
			CRP	mg/L	< 5

ACD = Anemia of chronic disease
TfS = Transferrin saturation
sTfR = soluble-Transferrin receptor
Hb = Hemoglobin
CRP = C-reactives protein

Table 30: Recommendations for monitoring in ACD patients receiving rhEPO therapy

Diagnostic Parameter	Target Values	Frequency of Determination
Hemoglobin	10-12 g/dL	every 3 months
Hematocrit	30-36 %	
Reticulocyte production index (RPI)	> 2	
Folate	> 20 ng/mL	every 6 months
Vitamin B_{12}	> 2 ng/mL	
Ferritin (F)	100-300 ng/mL	At beginning of correction phase and every three months after end of correction phase
soluble transferrin Receptor (s-TfR)	< 5 mg/L	
Transferrin saturation	20-30 %	
Hypochromic erythrocytes	< 10 %	
CRP	< 5mg/L	

All hematological parameters and iron parameters should be determined after commencing therapy with rhEPO and i.v. iron. These parameters should be monitored four times a year.

Disturbances of Iron Utilization
Diagnosis and Therapy

In patients with disturbances of iron utilization, the individual erythrocyte contains a normal amount of hemoglobin despite the lowering of the patient's hemoglobin value. MCH and MCV are normal. Iron deficiency is apparently not the problem in this case, but rather the *erythrocyte balance* between formation and decomposition. This balance is reflected in the reticulocyte count (as a measure of the regeneration of erythropoiesis) with normal reticulocyte values between 5 and 15%.

- Normochromic and normoregenerative anemias are usually based on inadequate stimulation of erythropoiesis. In patients with renal anemia, erythropoietin synthesis is greatly reduced when chronic renal insufficiency is present.
- Increased reticulocyte production index values > 2 are measured in patients with *hyperregeneration*. It is the response to the increased decomposition of erythrocytes by hemolysis.
  When erythrocyte decomposition is elevated, haptoglobin is used as the transport protein for hemoglobin and it drops rapidly. Haptoglobin is therefore a marker for diagnosis of hemolysis. Bilirubin increases noticeably only in the presence of acute or relatively intense erythrocyte decomposition.
- Lowered reticulocyte production index values < 2 are measured primarily in the presence of *hyporegeneration*, i.e., hypoplasia or even aplasia in the bone marrow.

Uremic Anemia

Uremic anemia is an important special form of normochromic normocytic anemia.

The clinical finding that plasma erythropoietin is lower in uremic patients than in non-uremic patients with a comparable degree of anemia suggests that uremic anemia is caused by the inadequate production of erythropoietin by chronically diseased kidneys.

Although uremic anemia is obviously multifactorial in origin and can be partially improved by appropriate hemodialysis therapy, the role

Clinical Aspects

played by the extracorporeal hemolytic component must not be under-estimated. Many patients have developed a defect in the hexose mono-phosphatase shunt; in addition, influences in hemodialysis such as mechanical intravascular hemolysis or pump trauma play an increasing role.

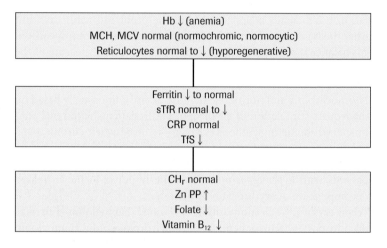

sTfR   =   soluble transferrin receptor
TfR   =   Transferrin saturation
CRP   =   C-reactive protein
CHr   =   hemoglobin content of reticulocytes
Zn PP =   zinc protoporphyrin

**Fig. 45: Laboratory findings of in patients with uremic anemia without EPO
        therapy**

The concentrations of the transferrin receptors in the plasma are lower than in healthy subjects when ferritin depots are adequate [55, 87].

This is not surprising if we bear in mind that the main production centers of the transferrin receptor are the immature cells of erythro-poiesis, which are reduced in mass in chronic renal failure. Therefore it would appear that serum transferrin receptor production in renal ane-mias is also dependent on erythropoietin [55, 87].

Remarkably, uremic anemia is well tolerated by patients and hemo-globin values up to 5 g/dl are well tolerated without side effects. In most patients the reticulocyte count is low and the survival time of blood cells is only moderately decreased. Anemia is thus the result of a massively disturbed erythrocyte production in the bone marrow.

If there are adequate ferritin depots, uremic anemia can be slightly improved by hemodialysis. A successful kidney transplant is the only way to achieve full correction, however.

Since the folic acid and vitamin B_{12} deficiency in dialysis patients can contribute to the development of anemia, care should be taken to maintain sufficiently high depot iron reserves and to avoid a folic acid deficit.

Indication of Iron Replacement

Ferritin should be determined upon commencement of treatment with rhEPO. In order to obtain an optimal therapeutic response to rhEPO, the serum ferritin level should exceed 100 mg/L. The loading of the iron stores should be checked using ferritin determinations performed many times throughout the year in order to exclude iron deficiency and iron overload in patients on parenteral iron replacement therapy.

In case of an inadequate response to rhEPO, the causes are to be excluded (Tab. 31).

Table 31: Causes of reduced response to rhEPO in patients with uremic anemia

Absolute iron deficiency	• Ferritin < 100 µg/L TfS < 20 %
Functional iron deficiency	• Ferritin > 100 µg/L TfS < 20 %
Bloodloss	
Infection, inflammation	• Leukocytes, CRP
Malignancies	
Medications	• ACs inhibitors and angiotensin II in high doses • Cyclosphosphamide • Azathioprin

If function iron deficiency exists, determination of the hypochromic erythrocytes is often helpful. If the portion of this erythrocyte subpopulation is above 10%, parenteral iron substitution will definitely improve the response of erythropoiesis to rhEPO. About 150 mg iron are required to raise hemoglobin by 1 g/dL. In order to correct hemoglobin by 3 – 4 g/dL, therefore, 450 – 600 mg iron are required for hemoglobin synthesis. Hemolysis patients require increased doses of iron, e.g., about 2 – 3 g per year, for the duration of erythropoietin treatment due to the loss of blood incurred in the course of treatment. Such amounts of iron typically must be administered parenterally, as the majority of patients do not tolerate higher doses of oral iron therapy due to intestinal side-effects. The risk of an iatrogenic iron overload during long-term replacement with parenteral iron is minimal as long as ferritin is monitored regularly.

Anaphylactoidal reactions of the type described in the context of ferric dextran – still widely used in the United States – are rare occurrences when Ferrlecit® or Venofer® are used [85, 86].

Therapy of Uremic Anemia

Patients with chronic renal insufficiency, including those on chronic hemodialysis (CHD) and frequent blood transfusions are favorite candidates for rhEPO therapy.

The rapidity and extent of the hematocrit increase are regulated by the rhEPO dose. Poor response can be caused by an iron deficiency due to inadequate iron stores or deficient mobilization from these stores (functional iron deficiency). An increasing hypochromia of erythrocytes and reticulocytes is often an early indicator of this, as the amount of iron available for Hb synthesis is inadequate.

Further causes of a diminished ability to respond to rhEPO are a vitamin deficiency (B_{12}, folic acid) or a reduction in stem cells in the bone marrow in patients with secondary hyperparathyroidism.

The difficulty of successful therapy of renal anemia, however, is to correct the transport iron deficiency and avoid a significant iron overload. Transferrin saturation should be significantly more than 20% and storage iron levels should exceed 100 ng/ml of ferritin, if absolute or functional iron deficiency as the cause of an inadequate therapeutic response to recombinant erythropoietin (rhEPO) is to be excluded.

Table 32: Objectives for the iron metabolism of dialysis patients undergoing erythropoietin and i.v. iron therapy

---

- Replacement of any depot iron deficiency (rare)

  Objective: 100 µg/L ≥ Ferritin ≤ 400 µg/L

- Treatment of a transport iron deficiency (frequent, due to iron mobilization disturbances)

  Objective: 15 % ≥ transferrin saturation ≤ 45 %

- Avoidance of a significant iron overload

  Warning limits: Tf saturation   > 45 %

  sTfR   < 5 mg/L

  Ferritin   > 400 µg/L

  CRP   > 5 mg/L

Low serum ferritin values (less than 100 ng/ml) in patients with uremia signify an absolute iron deficiency. High ferritin values, however, do not completely exclude functional iron deficiency.

Functional iron deficiency is characterized by normal (100-400 mg/L) or elevated (above 400 mg/L) ferritin values as well as reduced transferrin saturation values (less than 20%) and elevated sTfR values.

Criteria for a sufficient supply of iron are a ferritin level of at least 100 mg/L and a transferrin saturation of more than 20%. The soluble transferrin receptor concentration should be less than 5 mg/L (values are dependent on the method used) [103].

If dialysis patients do not meet these criteria, then 10 mg of iron per dialysis should be administered after replenishing the iron depot to a ferritin level of 100 mg/L. In non-dialysis patients oral iron replacement may be adequate (100 to 300 mg/day of iron(II)).

The therapeutic aim is to increase the hemoglobin concentration to 11-13 g/dL. The total iron requirement can be estimated using the following simple formula [85, 121, 167]:

Iron requirement (mg) = 150 mg x (HB1-Hb0)

Hb0 is the initial hemoglobin concentration, and Hb1 is the target hemoglobin concentration.

This formula provides a good estimation. For cases of extreme anemia, however, use Cook's equation (Fig. 46).

The target values are listed in Table 33.

Ferritin values of over 400 mg/L should be avoided in the long term on account of the concomitant danger of iron deposits forming outside the reticuloendothelial system. If values exceed this threshold during intravenous therapy, then a break in the therapy for a period of 3 months should be considered but erythropoietin treatment should be continued. The danger of iron overload in the context of parenteral substitution therapy adapted to iron losses of approximately 1.0 – 1.5 g per year can be considered to be low for hemodialysis patients. In the maintenance phase a low-dose, high-frequency administration of iron (10 to a maximum of 20 mg iron saccharate per hemodialysis) is currently preferred.

Table 33: Preliminary recommendations for iron replacement in dialysis patients

Correction		Maintenance of Hb (ferritin) concentration	
EPO:	about 2000 IU/patient/dialysis with 3 dialysis per week		
i.v. iron	10 – 40 mg/week	i.v. iron	10 – 20 mg/week
Target Hb	10 – 12 g/dL	Hb	11 – 13 g/dL
Target ferritin	100 µg/L	Ferritin	< 400 µg/L
Target transferrin saturation (TfS)	15 – 45 %	Transferrin saturation(TfS) (will be replaced by TfR in future)	15 – 45 %
Target soluble transferrin receptor (sTfR)	< 5 mg/L	soluble transferrin receptor (sTfR)	< 5 mg/L
CRP concentration	< 5 mg/L	CRP concentration	< 5 mg/L

No acute phase reaction was detected in patients undergoing dialysis who were administered iron as shown by the determination of CRP, IL-6 (interleukin-6), orosomucoid (alpha 1-acid-glycoprotein) and SAA (serum-amyloid-A-protein). Possible side effects of long-term iron supplementation causing ferritin values to exceed 400 µg/L are: increased risk of infection, elevated risk of developing carcinomas and an increased cardiovascular risk [138, 173, 174].

Table 34: Recommendations for diagnosis in patients on hemodialysis undergoing rhEPO and i.v. iron therapy

Diagnostic Parameter	Target Values	Frequency of Determination
Hemoglobin (Hb)	10-12 g/dL	
Hematocrit (Hct, PVC)	35-50 %	
Hypochromic Erythrocytes	< 10 %	every 3 month
Hypochromic Reticulocyte (CHr)	10-15 ‰	
Reticulocyte production index (RPI)	> 2	
Folate	> 30 ng/mL	every 6 month
Vitamin B$_{12}$	> 3 ng/mL	
Ferritin (F)	100-400 µg/L	At beginning of correction phase
Transferrin saturation (TfS)	15-45 %	and every three months after
soluble transferrin Receptor (sTfR)	< 5 mg/L	end of correction phase
CRP	< 5mg/L	

After commencing with rhEPO therapy and approx. 3 weeks after the end of the correction phase with i.v. iron, all hematological parameters and iron parameters should be determined. These parameters should be monitored four times a year.

Iron overload should be avoided during rhEPO therapy with concomitant iron supplementation.

In the context of the therapy of uremic anemia, the erythropoietin doses administered should be matched to the individual needs of the patient because the amount required by the uremic patient can be subject to considerable change. Provided iron reserves are sufficient, however, it is much lower than previously assumed. The erythropoietin dose can be significantly reduced in dialysis patients receiving optimized intravenous iron therapy. Hörl reported a reduction in the mean EPO dosage from 220 to 60 U/kg/week, and Schäfer reported a reduction from 140 to 70 U/kg/week [85].

The often discussed question of whether the dosage of erythropoietin is influenced by the route of administration is best answered by pointing out that, on parenteral iron therapy, there is no significant difference in the amount of erythropoietin required by intravenous and by subcutaneous administration. Similar observations were made by Sunder-Plasmann, Hörl and Taylor [85, 176].

Cook et al [35] as well as Mercuriali et al [131] have developed a therapeutic regimen for hemodialysis patients receiving rhEPO in which the targets are 100 mg/L serum ferritin and a transferrin saturation of

Clinical Aspects

more than 20% in order to ensure provision of adequate amounts of iron without the risk of iron overload.

How much iron should be administered to achieve a target value of 100 mg/L ferritin?

To guarantee optimal patient care for patients receiving rhEPO in combination with i.v. Fe (III) injections, body iron store parameters (see Fig. 46) should be determined at regular intervals.

These recommendations are summarized in Fig. 46.

$$\text{i.v. Iron (mg)} = 880 - 400 \text{ x (ln OF} - 2.4)$$
$$\text{ln OF} = \text{log natural of observed ferritin}$$

ln OF =   log natural of observed ferritin
ln 2.4 =   log natural of serum ferritin value
            of 12 mg/L

Example: observed serum ferritin value OF = 50 μg/L

ln OF = 3.9

$$
\begin{aligned}
\text{i.v. iron amount in (mg)} \ &= 880 - 400 \text{ x } (3.9 - 2.4) \\
&= 880 - 400 \text{ x } 1.5 \\
&= 880 - 600 \\
&= 280 \text{ mg}
\end{aligned}
$$

280 mg of i.v. iron are required to increase the ferritin level of the dialysis patient from 50 μg/L to 100 μg/L. This should be achieved in 10 dialysis sessions, i.e., within 3 to 4 weeks.

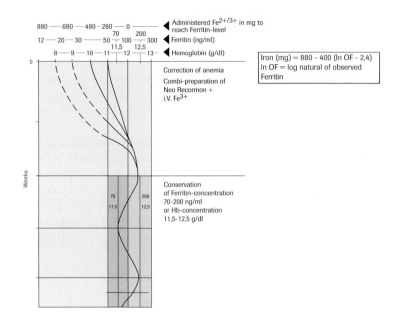

Iron (mg) = 880 - 400 (ln OF - 2,4)
ln OF = log natural of observed Ferritin

Fig. 46: **Cook's equation for determining iron dosage in patients with renal anemia. Using a nomogram, it is possible to calculate the amount of iron required to achieve a target value of 100 ng/ml ferritin and 12 g/l hemoglobin while maintaining administration of erythropoietin constant.**
(Cook, JD et al. (1986) [37] and Mercuriali, F. et al. (1994) [131])

Iron Overload

The human body is incapable of actively excreting excess iron. An over-abundant supply of iron leads to increased concentrations of the iron storage proteins ferritin and hemosiderin. If the storage capacity is exceeded, deposition takes place in the parenchymatous organs. The resulting cell damage leads to cell death and to functional impairment of the organ in question.

It has been suggested that this damage is due to toxic effects of free iron ions on the enzyme metabolism and to lysosome damage.

Iron overload, unlike iron deficiency, is rare. However, it is often overlooked or misinterpreted, and can progress to a life-threatening stage as a result. An elevated ferritin level should always suggest an iron overload, and the possibility of a true iron overload should be explored by differential diagnosis. On the other hand, disturbances of iron distribution must also be considered as a possibility (Tab. 35).

Representative Ferritin Increase

Iron storage diseases can be divided into a primary HLA-associated form, known as idiopathic hemochromatosis, and various secondary forms, or acquired hemochromatoses. The secondary forms are also known as hemosideroses.

Table 35: Causes of iron overload

1. Primary, hereditary hemochromatosis (HLA associated)
2. Secondary acquired hemochromatosis
• Ineffective erythropoiesis
- Thalassemia major
- Sideroblastic anemias
- Aplastic anemias
• Transfusion
3. Diet-related hemochromatosis
• Excessive iron intake
- Bantusiderosis (partially)
- Chronic alcoholism

HLA = human leucocyte antigen

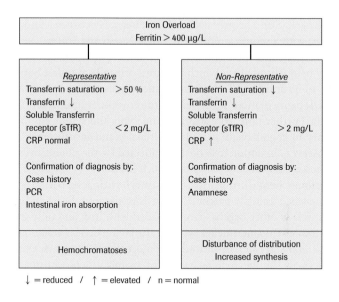

| Iron Overload |
| Ferritin > 400 µg/L |

Representative	Non-Representative
Transferrin saturation > 50 %	Transferrin saturation ↓
Transferrin ↓	Transferrin ↓
Soluble Transferrin receptor (sTfR) < 2 mg/L	Soluble Transferrin receptor (sTfR) > 2 mg/L
CRP normal	CRP ↑
Confirmation of diagnosis by: Case history PCR Intestinal iron absorption	Confirmation of diagnosis by: Case history Anamnese
Hemochromatoses	Disturbance of distribution Increased synthesis

↓ = reduced / ↑ = elevated / n = normal

Fig. 47: Differential diagnosis of clinical pictures with elevated ferritin levels

Primary Hemochromatosis

In primary hereditary HLA-associated hemochromatosis, an autosomal recessive disturbance of iron metabolism is apparent which can lead to severe parenchymal iron overload. The genetic defect is situated in a gene mutation on the short arm of chromosome 6 (HFE gene) and causes increased iron absorption in the small intestine and increased storage in the affected organs, namely the parenchymal cells of the liver, the heart, the pancreas, and the adrenal glands with the appropriate accompanying clinical complications such as diabetes, cirrhosis of the liver, arthropathy, cardiomyopathy and impotence.

The transport protein for iron, DTC 1, is mainly localized in the duodenum within the enterocytic membrane and increases in concentration during alimentary iron deficiency. DTC 1 is also expressed in the kidneys, liver, brain and heart [70]. The HFE genetic product - which is responsible for increased absorption of iron - is localized in the gastrointestinal tract and in the mutated form it is not capable of migrating

Clinical Aspects

out of the cell [56]. The prevalence of the disease is between 4 and 14% in Europe with a significant divide between North and South.

Men are affected approximately 10 times more often than women by primary hemochromatosis which becomes clinically manifest between the ages of 35 and 55 and causes liver function disorders, diabetes mellitus, dark pigmentation of the skin, cardiomyopathy and resulting arrhythmia. Furthermore, complaints of the joints and symptoms due to secondary hypogonadism as well as adrenal gland insufficiency have been observed. In about 15% of those affected by the illness, liver cell carcinoma arises, which represents a 300-fold risk.

In primary hemochromatosis, the plasma ferritin level rises at a relatively late stage. Initially parenchymal cells of the liver, heart and pancreas as well as other organs are overloaded with iron and only thereafter is the reticuloendothelial system saturated. Ferritin values above 400 mg/L and a transferrin saturation of more than 50% signify existing iron overload. In the manifest stage of primary hemochromatosis, ferritin concentrations in serum are usually over 700 mg/L. Transferrin is almost completely saturated.

Liver biopsy was the most appropriate in the past to conclusively diagnose primary hyperchromatosis, but a major advance has been made recently by the advent of identifying specific genetic changes for diagnosing the disease. The genetic defect can be identified using a molecular biological test. Hemochromatosis can be identified in 80% of the cases using the simple and relatively economically feasible PCR and DNA sequencing technologies before the manifestation of clinical symptoms. This opens up the possibility of timely treatment such that late-stage complications like cirrhosis of the liver and cancer of the liver can be prevented.

As was the case in the past, the therapy of choice is still phlebotomy. The aim of the therapy is to deplete iron stores as much as possible. The determination of the body iron status should be performed frequently at short intervals and in hereditary hemochromatosis the determination of plasma ferritin has proven to be of worth. The progression of the clinical parameter determines the necessity of continuing phlebotomy therapy. Phlebotomy at weekly, monthly or quarterly intervals may be necessary, however the therapy should never completely cease. As described above, the aim of phlebotomy is to prevent a negative progression of the disease.

Early identification of patients at risk which has become possible by virtue of the molecular biological detection of genetic defects can probably drastically reduce the incidence of hepatocellular carcinomas. Careful monitoring is required using imaging procedures (sonography, computer tomography [CT], nuclear magnetic resonance [NMR]), and regular determination of the a-fetoprotein (AFP).

Secondary Hemochromatosis

Hematopoietic disorders with concomitant ineffective or hypoplastic erythropoiesis such as thalassemia major, sideroblastic anemia or aplastic anemia are considered to be secondary or acquired hemochromatoses. In contrast to primary hemochromatosis in the secondary form the cells of the reticuloendothelial system are initially overloaded with iron. Organ damage occurs at a relatively late stage. They arise because of a redistribution of iron from the cells of the reticuloendothelial system into parenchymal cells of individual organs. The duration of chronic iron overloading in secondary iron storage disorders is therefore a critical factor.

Acquired hemochromatoses can also develop from alimentary iron overload, parenteral administration of iron and transfusions or other chronic diseases with ineffective erythrocytopoiesis.

Alcoholics with chronic liver disease in whom iron deposits have been detected after liver biopsies but whose total body iron levels are within the non-pathological range present a particular diagnostic challenge. The body's total iron reserves are normal. Such patients probably suffer from an alcohol-induced liver disease (toxic nutritive cirrhosis) and seem to acquire iron deposits as a result of cell necroses and iron uptake from such necrotic cells.

However, a second group of alcoholics has been identified who have extremely high deposits of iron in their bodies and massive iron deposits in the cirrhotic liver. Such patients may suffer from congenital primary hemochromatosis with concomitant toxic nutritive liver disease. The molecular biological detection of causative primary hemochromatosis makes differential diagnosis more straight forward.

Patients suffering from renal insufficiency on dialysis were first treated with erythropoietin in 1988 and for this group of patients iron overloading caused by transfusions should belong firmly to the past.

Clinical Aspects

Non-iron-induced Disturbances of Erythropoiesis

Deficiencies in vitamin B_{12}, folic acid and/or erythropoietin have been found to be crucial factors in non-iron-deficiency-induced forms of anemia.

An initial diagnosis can be made with a high degree of accuracy by recording the patient's history or from knowledge of the primary disease. Given the known interaction between vitamin B_{12} and folic acid, the determination of these two cofactors by immunoassay should now be standard clinical practice. Sternal puncture or bone biopsies also offer clear histological and morphological pictures.

Deficiency in folic acid or vitamin B_{12} is the main feature of diseases accompanied by macrocytic anemia.

In the differential diagnosis of macrocytic anemia, an elevated level of LDH with simultaneous reticulocytosis and hyperbilirubinemia (both to be interpreted as hyperregeneratory anemia) directs attention to a vitamin B_{12} deficit. Macrocytic anemia without these components makes a genuine folic acid deficiency likely (pregnancy, alcohol).

Table 36: Deficiencies in the cofactors of erythropoiesis

Microcytic anemia	Macrocytic anemia	Normocytic anemia
Iron metabolism disturbances	Folic acid deficiency	Renal anemia (erythropoietin deficiency)
Hemoglobinopathies (e.g., thalassemia)	B_{12} deficiency Drug-induced	Hemolytic anemia
	Alcohol consumption	Hemoglobinopathies
	MDS	Bone marrow diseases
		Toxic bone marrow damage

MDS = myelodysplastic syndrome

Normocytic forms of anemia draw attention to the hemolytic component of erythrocyte destruction, with haptoglobin playing the crucial role as the key to diagnosis. Erythrocyte morphology provides a means to exclude mechanical hemolysis or to look for hemoglobinopathy (Hb electrophoresis) or an enzyme defect.

Proof of impaired renal function makes it likely that the most important deficiency of a cofactor in Hb synthesis is present, a deficiency of erythropoietin.

The determination of erythropoietin which can now be performed by immunoassay at least forms a good base for a prognosis of the outcome of treatment. Before giving any treatment with erythropoietin, it is important to determine the iron depots; otherwise, action by the parenterally administered erythropoietin, which is genetically engineered today, is impossible.

Macrocytic, Hyperchromic Anemia

Hyperchromic macrocytic anemias (MCH above 33 pg, MCV usually above 96 fl) and a typical blood count almost always indicate a vitamin deficiency of B_6, B_{12} or folic acid and normo- to hyporegeneratory (reticulocytes below 5%). In advanced stages, vitamin deficiency can also affect the remaining cell lines (leucocytopenia, thrombocytopenia). The most frequent cause of a hyperchromic anemia is chronic alcoholism.

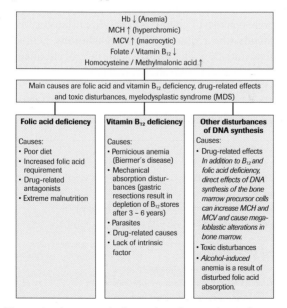

Fig. 48: Diagnosis of macrocytic, hyperchromic anemias and causes

A non-representative ferritin increase may indicate disturbances in the proliferation and maturation of bone marrow cells induced by vitamin deficiency.

These macrocytic forms of anemia are caused by disturbed DNA synthesis. As non-iron-induced disturbances of erythropoiesis, they influence not only the proliferation of cells of erythropoiesis, but above all that of the gastrointestinal epithelial cells. Since considerable numbers of macrocytic cells are destroyed while still in the bone marrow, they are also included under the heading ineffective erythropoiesis.

Most macrocytic forms of anemia are due to a deficiency in either vitamin B_{12} or folic acid, or both. The most common causes of folic acid and vitamin B_{12} deficiency are listed in Tables 37 and 38.

Drug-induced macrocytic anemia is now common. Drugs which disturb DNA synthesis are now part of the standard therapeutic armamentarium of chemotherapy (Tab. 32). There are also rare metabolic disturbances which cause macrocytic anemia, plus megaloblastic anemia with as yet unknown causes, such as the congenital dyserythropoietic anemias or anemias as part of the Di-Guglielmo syndrome (Tab. 37 and Tab. 38).

Acute severe macrocytic anemia is a rarity; it can be observed in intensive care patients who require multiple transfusions, hemodialysis or total parenteral nutrition. This form of acute macrocytic anemia may be limited mainly to patients who already had borderline folic acid depots before they fell ill.

Table 37: Drug-induced forms of macrocytic anemia

1. Drugs which act via folic acid
Malabsorption
– alcohol, phenytoin, barbiturates
Metabolism
– alcohol, methotrexate, pyrimethamine, triamterene, pentamidine
2. Drugs which act via vitamin B_{12}
PAS, colchicine, neomycin
3. Inhibitors of DNA metabolism
Purine antagonists (azathioprine, 6-mercaptopurine)
Pyrimidine antagonists (5-fluorouracil, cytosine arabinoside)
Others (procarbazine, acyclovir, zidovudine, hydroxyurea)

PAS = para-aminosalicylic acid

Clinical Aspects

Table 38: Symptomatic forms of macrocytic anemia

1. Metabolic diseases
  Aciduria (orotic acid)
2. Uncertain origin
  Di-Guglielmo syndrome
  Congenital dyserythropoietic anemia
  Refractory megaloblastic anemia

Folic Acid

Folic acid is reduced to tetrahydrofolic acid (THF) in the organism under the influence of ascorbic acid and vitamin B_{12}. As a transporter of activated C-1 groups (methyl-, formyl-, formiate- and hydroxymethyl groups), tetrahydrofolic acid performs an important function in amino acid and nucleotide metabolism and in the methylation of homocysteine to methionine. Folic acid is essential for the biosynthesis of purines and pyrimidines for DNA and RNA synthesis and, therefore, for all growth and cellular division processes. Since the erythropoietic cells of the bone marrow have high rates of cellular division, they are particularly dependent on an adequate supply of folic acid.

Requirement:
The body's total folic acid reserves are approximately 5 to 10 mg.

The German Society for Nutrition recommends a daily intake of 400 mg folic acid (dietary folate). The recommendation for women who are pregnant or breast-feeding is 600 mg folic acid (dietary folate) / day.

Due to the poor dietary intake of folic acid, certain basic foodstuffs (breakfast cereals, flour) have been enriched with folic acid in the United States since 1998.

The National Research Council of the United States recommends a daily dietary allowance of folic acid of 400 mg for adults up to 55 years of age. For adults above 55 years of age, the recommended dietary allowance (RDA) is 800 mg – 1200 mg/day.

Clinical Aspects

Table 39: Causes of Folic Acid Deficiency

1. Inadequate intake
Alcoholism
Unbalanced diet
2. Increased requirement
Pregnancy
Adolescence
Malignancy
Increased cell turnover (hemolysis, chronic exfoliative skin diseases)
Hemodialysis patients
3. Malabsorption
Sprue
Drugs (barbiturates, phenytoin)
4. Disturbed folic acid metabolism
Inhibition of dihydrofolic acid reductase (e.g., methotrexate, pyrimethamin, triamterene)
Congenital enzyme defects

Deficiency:

Patients with a folic acid deficit are usually in a poor nutritional state, and often have a range of gastrointestinal symptoms such as diarrhea, cheilosis and glossitis. In contrast to advanced vitamin B_{12} deficiency, no neurological deficits are found.

Folic acid deficiency can be attributed to three main causes: inadequate intake, increased requirement, and malabsorption.

Special attention must be devoted to various groups in the population who commonly have inadequate folic acid intake: chronic alcoholics, the elderly, and adolescents.

In chronic alcoholics, the alcohol (beer and wine) which is the main source of energy contains practically no folic acid or only small quantities. Alcohol also leads to disturbances in the processing of absorbed folic acid.

The folic acid deficit in the elderly seems to be caused mainly by an extremely unbalanced diet.

Unbalanced diets have a considerable attraction for adolescents. Those who consume fast food are particularly at risk.

An increased folic acid requirement is present during the growth phase in childhood and adolescence, as well as during pregnancy.

Investigations of elderly patients with hyperhomocysteinanemia but no traces of anemia make it necessary to correct the reference interval upward.

Clinical Aspects

Since the bone marrow and the intestinal mucosa have an increased folic acid requirement because of a high cell proliferation rate, patients with hematological diseases, especially those with increased erythropoiesis, may not be able to meet their increased folic acid requirement from their dietary intake.

Disturbances in the absorption of folic acid occur in both tropical sprue and gluten enteropathy. Manifest macrocytic anemia may develop in both clinical pictures. Other signs of malabsorption may also occur. Alcohol-induced folic acid deficiency may to a certain extent also be caused by malabsorption. Diseases of the small intestine may also prevent the absorption of folic acid. The folic acid absorption test is used as a general, practical means for detecting malabsorption.

Resorption Test:

The patient is given 1 mg folic acid i. v. or i. m. per day on the 4 days preceding the examination. This serves to make up any folic acid deficiency in the tissue which could affect the absorption test and produce a false positive result (no measurable increase in the serum folic acid concentration after oral ingestion). On the day of the examination the fasting patient is given 40 mg/kg folic acid orally, and the serum folic acid concentration is determined at the following times: 0, 60, 120 minutes. In normal patients the serum concentration rises to over 7 mg/L.

Folic acid is absorbed in the entire small intestine, so that the substance is suitable for a global test of small-intestine absorption. Data on normal serum concentrations vary slightly from laboratory to laboratory, but do not diverge to any great extent (0.19 – 0.96 mg/mL) [45]. Recent findings by Brouwer [24] and Hermann [81], however, suggest that the reference range should be corrected.

Therapy:

Low levels of folic acid in the serum or in the erythrocytes are a definite indication of folic acid deficiency. This condition is treated by oral replacement therapy, with 1 mg folic acid being administered daily. The reaction to the replacement therapy is similar to that in B_{12} deficiency, i.e. within 5 to 7 days there is an increase in the number of reticulocytes and the blood count returns to normal within 2 to 3 months.

Due to the disturbed development of erythrocyte, a deficiency of folic acid or vitamin B_{12} can lead to the formation of a macrocytic or megaloblastic anemia. Cell division in the erythropoietic cells in the bone marrow is slowed, so that megalocytes, instead of normal erythrocytes (normocytes), are formed. Megalocytes contain too much hemoglobin as compared to normal red blood cells.

To prevent neural tube defects, women who desire to become pregnant are recommended to begin early replacement of 0.4 to 0.8 mg folic acid per day.

Folic acid replacement can mask a deficiency of vitamin B_{12} (secondary folic acid deficiency in patients with pernicious anemia). Vitamin B_{12} returns N-methyl-tetrahydrofolic acid to tetrahydrofolic acid, which is important for DNA synthesis. Although inhibition of this conversion by vitamin B_{12} deficiency can be compensated by administering folic acid, the danger of severe neurological damage remains. The main cause of folic acid deficiency is an inadequate supply in the food (alcoholism, unbalanced diets, drugs). If these factors are not present in the patient's history, a B_{12} deficiency should also be ruled out.

Vitamin B_{12} Deficiency

Vitamin B_{12} (cyanocobalamin) is metabolized in the liver into the coenzymatically active forms 5'-deoxyadenosyl-cobalamin and methylcobalamin. These substances are involved in the biosynthesis of purine and pyrimidine bases, the synthesis of methionine from homocysteine, in the regeneration of N-methyl-tetrahydrofolic acid (secondary folic acid deficiency in patients with pernicious anemia) and the formation of myelin sheaths in the nervous system. Vitamin B_{12}, as well as folic acid, is involved in DNA synthesis and, consequently, has a strong influence on all cell division and growth processes.

Absorption of physiological doses takes place via an active absorption mechanism. To be absorbed in the intestine, Vitamin B_{12} ("extrinsic factor") requires the "intrinsic factor", a glycoprotein formed in the gastric mucosa.

Requirement:
The symptoms of vitamin B_{12} deficiency are partly hematological, partly gastroenterological. Neurological manifestations are often observed independently of the duration of vitamin B_{12} deficiency [88].

The hematological symptoms are almost always caused by an anemia. They include paleness, weakness, dizziness, tinnitus as well as coronary heart disease and myocardial insufficiency.

There is usually tachycardia with an enlarged heart; the liver and spleen may also be slightly enlarged. Fissures in the mucous membrane, a red tongue, anorexia, weight loss and occasional diarrhea indicate that the gastrointestinal system is involved.

It may be very difficult to classify the neurological symptoms. Irrespective of the duration of the vitamin B_{12} deficit, in extreme cases they may range from demyelinization to neuron death. The earliest neurological manifestations consist of paresthesia, but also weakness, ataxia and disturbances of fine coordination. Objectively, disturbance of deep sensibility usually occurs early and Rhomberg and Babinski are positive. The CNS symptoms range from forgetfulness to severe forms of dementia or psychoses. These neurological conditions may long precede the hematological manifestations, but as a rule hematological symptoms predominate in the average patient.

The main cause of vitamin B_{12} deficiency, the pernicious anemia, is a deficiency of intrinsic factor. It is generally accompanied by atrophy of the gastric mucosa.

Table 40: Causes of vitamin B_{12} deficiency

1. Inadequate intake
   Vegetarians (rare)
2. Malabsorption
   Deficiency of intrinsic factor
   - pernicious anemia
   - gastrectomy
   - congenital (extremely rare)
   Diseases of the terminal ileum
   - Sprue
   - Crohn's disease
   - Extensive resections
   - Selective malabsorption (Imerslund syndrome-extremely rare)
   Parasite-induced deficiencies
   - Fish tapeworm
   - Bacteria ("blind loop syndrome")
   Drug-induced
   - PAS, neomycin

PAS = para-aminosalicylic acid

Clinical Aspects

The disease shows geographical clustering in Northern Europe. It is generally a disease affecting the elderly beyond the age of 60; it is less common in children younger than 10 years old. It is found with striking frequency in black patients.

The current view about the pathogenesis of pernicious anemia is that it is produced by an autoimmune process directed against the parietal cells of the stomach. It is therefore most marked in patients with clinical pictures attributed to autoimmune diseases, such as immune hyperthyroidism, myxedema, idiopathic adrenal insufficiency, vitiligo and hypoparathyroidism. Antibodies against parietal cells can be detected in 90% of patients with pernicious anemia. The detection of these antibodies does not however mean that the pernicious anemia is necessarily manifest. The incidence of antibodies to intrinsic factor is about 60%.

Given the pathological mechanism involved, hypoacidity or anacidity is the rule, patients often have gastric polyps, and the incidence of stomach cancer doubles that in the normal population. If the source of the intrinsic factor is destroyed such as by total gastrectomy or by extensive destruction of the gastric mucosa (for example by corrosion) megaloblastic anemia may develop.

It should also not be forgotten that a number of bacteria in the intestinal flora require vitamin B_{12}. Deficiency syndromes may thus develop after anatomical lesions as a result of massive bacterial proliferation. Deficiency symptoms may also occur as a result of strictures, diverticula and the blind loop syndrome. They may also occur with pseudo obstruction in diabetes mellitus as a result of amyloid deposits, or in scleroderma. Vitamin B_{12}-deficiency anemia is also known to occur as a result of tropical sprue and the fish tapeworm. Most of these clinical pictures are also accompanied by malabsorption syndromes, often with steatorrhea.

Regional enteritis, Whipple's disease and tuberculosis may be accompanied by disturbances of vitamin B_{12} absorption. This also applies to chronic pancreatitis, in rare instances to Zollinger-Ellison syndrome and segmental diseases of the ileum [157].

Defects of absorption of vitamin B_{12} used to be detected by the Schilling Test. This test has been replaced by determination of parietal cell antibodies and antibodies against intrinsic factor.

Hereditary megaloblastic anemia is extremely rare; it is caused by congenital disturbances of orotic acid metabolism or, in Lesch-Nyhan syndrome, by the disturbance of enzymes involved in folic acid metabolism.

Therapy:

The most frequent cause of B_{12} deficiency is a lack of intrinsic factor, as in pernicious anemia or after a total gastrectomy. Reduced absorption in the ileum after extensive surgical resection or in Crohn's disease may also be a cause. All other causes have little practical relevance. Vitamin B_{12} must therefore be administered parenterally.

On account of the neurological and neuropsychiatric syndromes, which may also occur without blood count changes, and which are only then are definitely reversible if they have been present for less than 6 months, an initial high-dose treatment regimen has become established. This is a stepped regimen, in which 200 µg vitamin B_{12} is administered intramuscularly daily during the first week of therapy, followed by one intramuscular injection per week for 1 month and then monthly i.m. administration of 200 µg for the rest of the patient's life. It should be pointed out again that pernicious anemia is a life-long disease and that if the monthly treatment is interrupted, inevitably a vitamin deficiency will develop.

Clinical improvement is usually seen immediately after administration of vitamin B_{12}. Between the 5th and 7th day, if there are sufficient iron reserves, the so-called reticulocytic crisis appears and within 2 months the peripheral blood count has returned to normal. The CNS symptoms and their neurological manifestations return to normal as well.

Normochromic, Normocytic Anemia

If the individual erythrocyte contains a normal amount of hemoglobin (MCH 28 – 33 pg/cell) despite the lowering of the patient's hemoglobin value, then iron deficiency is apparently not the problem in this case, but rather the erythrocyte balance between formation and decomposition. This balance is reflected in the reticulocyte count:

• Increased reticulocyte counts (> 15%) are measured in patients with hyperregeneration. It is the response to the increased decomposition of erythrocytes = hemolysis.

Clinical Aspects

- Lowered reticulocyte counts are measured primarily in the presence of hyporegeneration, i.e., hypoplasia or even aplasia in the bone marrow.
- When erythrocyte decomposition is elevated, haptoglobin is used as the transport protein for hemoglobin and it drops rapidly. Haptoglobin is therefore a marker for hemolysis. Bilirubin increases noticeably only in the presence of acute or relatively intense erythrocyte decomposition (hemolysis). Normal haptoglobin values indicate the absence of hemolysis.

Normocytic anemia generally occurs during acute blood loss, in hemolysis and as a result of renal failure or endocrine disturbances.

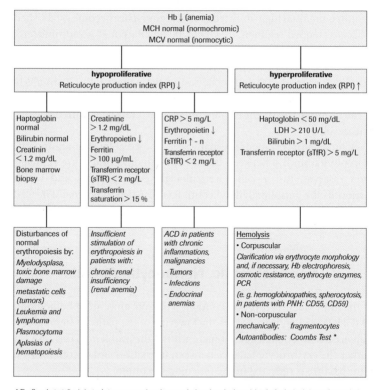

* The Coombs test discriminates between serogenic and corpuscular hemolyses by determining the freely circulating erythrocyte antibodies. The antibodies bound to erythrocytes are also determined indirectly. Most of the acquired hemolyses are <coombs positive>

Fig. 49: Diagnosis and causes of normochromic, normocytic anemia

Besides the formal pathological classification of anemia into microcytic, macrocytic and normocytic, differentiation by origin has now become established, especially in disturbances of erythropoiesis. The hemolytic anemias (cell trauma, membrane abnormality), enzyme disturbances (glucose-6-phosphate-dehydrogenase defect) and disturbances of hemoglobin synthesis have become clinically the most important.

Extracorpuscular Hemolytic Anemias

Hemolytic anemia is generally an acquired autoimmune hemolytic anemia. A common form of differentiation is based on the thermal behavior of the antibodies, as warm or cold antibodies.

The most common clinical pictures of symptomatic hemolytic anemia are summarized in Table 41.

Table 41: Antibody-induced hemolytic anemia

1. Warm antibodies

   Idiopathic
   Lymphomas
   Other neoplasms (rare)
   SLE (systemic lupus erythrematodes)
   Drugs

2. Cold antibodies

   Cold agglutinins
   - Infections (generally acute)
   - Lymphoma
   - Idiopathic
   Paroxysmal cold hemoglobinuria

3. Alloantibodies

   Blood transfusions
   Pregnancies

In the detection of hemolysis, the determination of haptoglobin and LDH in particular have proved to be diagnostically useful tests. After the occurrence of intravascular hemolysis, the haptoglobin concentration drops rapidly. This is attributable to the very short half-life of the haptoglobin-hemoglobin complex of only about 8 minutes. In its function as a transport (and acute-phase) protein it binds intravascular, free hemo-

Clinical Aspects

globin and transports it extremely rapidly to the reticulo-endothelial system for degradation.

Haptoglobin is therefore eminently suitable for the detection of hemolysis, i.e., for the diagnosis and assessment of the course of hemolytic diseases. Sharply decreased haptoglobin levels indicate intravascular hemolysis which may have immunohemolytic, microangiopathic, mechanical, drug (G-6-P-dehydrogenase deficiency) or infectious causes (e.g., malaria). Extravascular hemolysis (e.g., ineffective erythropoiesis, hypersplenism), on the other hand, shows a drop in haptoglobin only in hemolytic crises. Reduced haptoglobin levels may also be congenital (albeit rarely in Europe). They may also be observed in other, non-hemolytic diseases, e.g. in liver diseases and in malabsorption syndrome. Since the LDH concentration in the erythrocytes is about 360 times higher than in the plasma, with hemolytic processes there is a rise in LDH. The LDH increase stands in direct relationship to the erythrocyte destruction. A particularly large rise in LDH can be observed in hemolytic crises. Hemolytic anemia caused by a circulatory trauma is characterized by the occurrence of burr and helmet cells.

The most important clinical occurrences are listed in Table 42.

Table 42: Mechanically induced forms of hemolytic anemia

1. Microangiopathies

   Splenomegaly
   Hemolytic-uremic syndrome (HUS)
   Thrombotic-thrombocytopenic purpura (TTP)
   Cirrhosis of the liver
   Eclampsia

2. Prosthetic heart valves

3. Extracorporeal pump systems

   Hemodialysis
   Hemofiltration
   Extracorporeal oxygenation

Corpuscular Anemias

The most important of the enzyme defects is glucose-6-phosphate dehydrogenase deficiency with all its genetically fixed variants, of which favism is now clinically the best known form.

The hemoglobinopathy that has attained most importance is sickle-cell anemia in all its variants; Met-hemoglobin (met-Hb) is also worthy of mention as the cause of familiar cyanosis. The hemoglobinopathies also include all variants of thalassemia, a disorder which is gaining importance with the increasing mobility of the world's population. These hemoglobinopathies generally present a variable morphological picture with target cells. A clear diagnosis can be made only by hemoglobin electrophoresis or by high-pressure liquid chromatography (HPLC).

Influence of Erythropoiesis in Other Diseases

Erythropoietin is used successfully in patients with disturbances of iron utilization and distribution, chronic diseases and to promote erythropoiesis in individuals donating blood for their own use in planned orthopedic surgery.

Beginning just a few years ago, EPO has been produced using recombinant genetic engineering techniques. When expressed in mammalian cells, EPO receives the necessary high portion of carbohydrates. The half life of intravenously administered EPO is about 5 hours [69].

A very successful therapy with erythropoietin is used with anemic AIDS patients. In patients with hemoblastoses and malignancies on chemotherapy, the suppression of erythropoiesis - which is often a result of intensive chemotherapy - can be overcome with erythropoietin therapy.

A new therapeutic strategy using EPO has been used successfully in treating anemic newborns. Due to the relative hypoxia during intrauterine growth, newborns have a polycythemia. In adapting to the environmental conditions, erythropoiesis is slowed greatly after birth. The reduced erythropoiesis leads to physiological anemia in newborns after 8 to 12 weeks. After that, the level of erythropoietin rises once more, and erythropoiesis reaches a normal level. Symptoms of anemia are rarely observed in mature newborns, although aggravating factors occur with premature infants. The number of erythrocytes is lower at birth than in mature newborns, and their erythrocyte life span is shorter. Premature infants therefore often tend to develop anemias.

Approximately 50% of all premature infants have an Hb concentration less than 9 g/dL. This development of anemia can be bridged by the administration of erythropoietin, and it can replace the transfusion therapy used in the past. Additional iron replacement is recommended.

Increasingly, autologous blood donations are being set aside by patients before they undergo a planned surgical procedure in order to avoid the risk of contracting HIV or hepatitis if they should require a blood transfusion. The risk of contracting an infection from a homologous conserved blood donation is about 1 : 1 million for an HIV infection, 1 : 50,000 for a hepatitis B infection, and 1 : 5,000 for a hepatitis C infection.

The indications for replacement therapy with erythropoietin are increasing, not only because they are free of side effects. The effectiveness of the therapy must be monitored at all times, however, in order to determine the response rate and to control the therapy. The changes in lipid metabolism on erythropoietin therapy are also worthy of mention. A significant decrease in serum cholesterol has been seen [104].

Clinical Aspects

Methods of Determination in Serum/Plasma and Blood

The methods of determination for plasma proteins, the blood count and for inflammation are only described in principle; the listed references allow the reader to obtain further and more detailed information. The recommended reference intervals apply only to the methods described in the respective references.

The development of new methods, the improvement of existing methods, high quality standards as well as increasing national and international standardization have resulted in an increase in the clinical sensitivity and specificity of clinical laboratory-diagnostic investigations. The current international standard is mentioned whenever possible.

Determination in Serum/Plasma

In addition to the blood count, hemoglobin and hematocrit, the search for disturbances in iron metabolism is based on a number of important investigation methods in serum and plasma:

- Iron
- Hemoglobin (Hb)
- Total iron binding capacity (TIBC)
- Latent iron binding capacity (LIBC)
- Ferritin
- Transferrin (Tf)
- Transferrin saturation (TfS)
- Soluble transferrin receptor (sTfR)
- Haptoglobin (Hp)
- Ceruloplasmin (Cp)
- Folic acid
- Vitamin B_{12}
- Erythropoietin (EPO)
- Homocysteine
- Methylmalonic acid

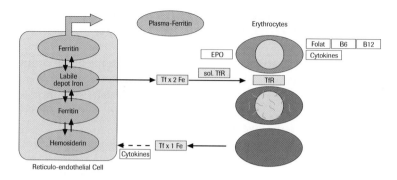

Fig. 50: Iron metabolism

Table 43: Concentration ranges of the analysis

Parameter	Reference concentration intervals for adults		Analytical method
	[µg/dL]	**[µmol/l]**	
Iron(Fe)	40-160	7-29*	Spectrophotometry
Hemoglobin (Hb)	$12 - 17 \times 10^6$ (12 – 17 g/dL)	$7.5 - 9 \times 10^3$ **	Spectrophotometry
Iron-binding capacity (TIBC)	260-500	46-90	Spectrophotometry
Transferrin (Tf)	200 000-400 000 (= 2-4 g/l)	25-50**	Immunochem. method
Soluble transferrin receptor (sTfR)	500-3000 (= 0.5-3 mg/L)	$6-35 \times 10^{-3}$ ****	Immunochem. method
Ferritin	1-30 (= 10-300 µg/L)	$0.2-7 \times 10^{-6}$ *****	Immunochem. method
Haptoglobin (Hp)	60 000-270 000 (= 0.6-2.7 g/dL)	$7-32^+$	Immunochem. method
Ceruloplasmin (Cp)	15 000-60 000	$1 - 5^{++}$	Immunochem. method
Folic acid	0.2-2 (=2-20 ng/mL)	$5-45 \times 10^{-3}$ $^{+++}$	Immunochem. method
Vitamin B_{12}	$20-90 \times 10^{-3}$	$150-670 \times 10^{-6}$ $^{++++}$	Immunochem. method
Erythropoietin (EPO)	6-25 U/l		Immunochem. method

*	Rel. atomic weight of iron:	56 Daltons		
**	Rel. atomic weight of hemoglobin	68 000 Daltons		
***	Rel. atomic weight of transferrin:	79 570 Daltons	(apotransferrin)	
****	Rel. atomic weight of soluble transferrin receptor:	85 000 Daltons		
*****	Rel. atomic weight of ferritin:	440 000 Daltons		
+	Rel. atomic weight of haptoglobin:	100 000 Daltons	Type	Hp 1-1
		200 000 Daltons		Hp 2-1
		400 000 Daltons		Hp 2-2
++	Rel. atomic weight of coeruloplasmin	132 000 Daltons		
+++	Rel. atomic weight of folic acid:	445 Daltons		
++++	Rel. atomic weight of vitamin B_{12}:	1355 Daltons		
+++++	Rel. atomic weight of erythropoietin:	34 000 Daltons		

Free iron ions do not occur in the blood. Plasma or serum iron is almost entirely transferrin-bound. Because of its technical simplicity, the determination of transferrin saturation (TfS) has displaced the determination of the iron-binding capacity. Due to the strong dependence of iron concentration on the circadian rhythm, the determination of the soluble transferrin receptor (sTfR) - which does not depend on these fluctuations - is carried out with increasing frequency in place of TfS. TfS is now required almost exclusively to diagnose hemochromatoses. Ferritin is the depot protein, which occurs not only intracellularly, but also (in very low concentrations) in the blood and is an index of size of the iron stores.

Iron

In addition to the colorimetric methods, which are by far the most commonly used, atomic absorption spectrophotometry (AAS) and potentiostatic coulometry are also available as special techniques. More than 95% of all iron determinations in clinical laboratories are performed colorimetrically, in most cases using routine analyzers.

All the colorimetric methods developed for the determination of iron have the following steps in common:
• *Liberation* of the Fe^{3+} ions from the transferrin complex by acids or tensides.

In some methods, the liberation of Fe^{3+} ions by acid is combined with deproteinization after addition of trichloroacetic acid or chloroform. Deproteinization is unnecessary if a suitable tenside (e.g., guanidinium chloride) is used in a weakly acidic solution (pH 5). The liberation of Fe^{3+} by a tenside without deproteinization has the advantages that there is no turbidity due to incomplete deproteinization, the removal of Fe^{3+} from the transferrin is complete, and hemoglobin-bound Fe^{2+} is not liberated.
• *Reduction* of Fe^{3+} ions to Fe^{2+} ions

To enable the color reaction with a suitable chromophore to take place, the Fe^{3+} ions must first be reduced. Ascorbate has proved to be a parti-

cularly suitable reducing agent; hydroquinone, thioglycolate, and hydroxylamine are also used.
• *Reaction* of the Fe^{2+} ions to form a color complex

The only complexing agents used nowadays are bathophenanthroline and Ferro Zine® (registered trade name, Hach Chemical Co., Ames, Iowa/USA). Ferro Zine has a higher extinction coefficient than bathophenanthroline and its solubility is also better. Slightly higher iron values are obtained with Ferro Zine.

At present there is no reference method for the determination of serum/plasma iron. However, reference methods have been proposed by the International Committee for Standardization in Hematology (ICSH) [88] and more recently by the Center of Disease Control (CDC).

The method recommended in 1972 by the ICSH uses 2 mol/l hydrochloric acid for the liberation of the Fe^{3+} ions and thioglycolic acid for the reduction. The complexing agent is bathophenanthroline-disulphonate.

The CDC proposal is a method with deproteinization by trichloroacetic acid, and with reduction by ascorbic acid. The complexing agent is Ferro Zine.

In the Ferro Zine method without deproteinization, the reaction is measured in the cuvette itself. The Ferro Zine iron complex formed can be measured in the wavelength range from 530 to 560 nm by any routine analyzer.

Table 44: Historical survey

Year	Milestone
1958	Bathophenanthroline method without deproteinization (Sanford und Ramsay)
1972	Bathophenanthroline method (ICSH recommendation)
1990	Ferro Zine method with deproteinization (CDC recommendation)
1998	Ferro Zine method without deproteinization

Every serum sample contains the five iron fractions listed in Table 45.

Table 45: Iron fractions

Fractions	Iron concentration in serum
Trivalent iron in transferrin	ca. 50-150 µg/dL Fe^{3+}
Divalent iron in hemoglobin	5-10 µg/dL Fe^{2+}
Trivalent iron in ferritin	0.2-10 µg/dL Fe^{3+}
Complexed iron	< 0.5 µg/dL Fe^{2+}/Fe^{3+}
Iron ions due to contamination	<< 0.5 µg/dL Fe^{3+}/Fe^{2+}

The iron level shows a distinct circadian rhythm. There is also a considerable day-to-day variation. Serum iron is protein-bound. The collection of blood samples must therefore be standardized with respect to time, body position and venous occlusion [Fig. 51].

Iron is one of the trace elements, with a concentration in the serum similar to those of copper and zinc. Contamination must therefore be avoided during the collection and preparation of samples.

Serum and heparinized plasma are suitable for use as samples. EDTA plasma cannot be used. Hemolysis interferes. No detectable change in the iron concentration is found upon storage of serum for several weeks at +4º C.

Reference range:
Reference range for serum/plasma iron in healthy subjects [75]:

Women	37-145 [mg/dL]	6.6-26 [mmol/l]
Men	59-158 [mg/dL]	11-28 [mmol/l]

Notes:
Considerable differences are found in the reference ranges given in the literature for iron. There are various reasons for this:

The reference range does not have a normal distribution.
• Iron concentrations found for men are about 15 to 20% higher than those for women.
• Iron concentrations are high in babies, but decrease from the 2nd to the 3rd year of life.

Laboratory

- The plasma iron level has a pronounced circadian rhythm. The difference between morning and evening values can be up to 50 mg/dL. Day-to-day and week-to-week variations in the same individual are also very pronounced (Fig. 52).

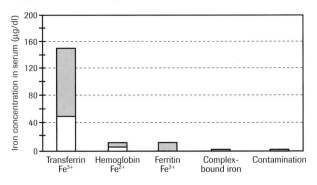

Fig. 51: Distribution of plasma iron

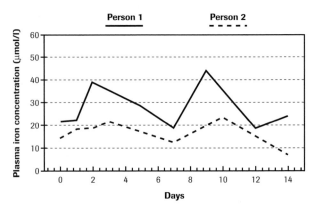

Fig. 52: Day to day fluctuations of the plasma iron concentration

Iron Saturation = Total Iron-Binding Capacity (TIBC) and Determination of the Latent Iron-Binding Capacity (LIBC)

These methods have now been largely replaced by the determination of transferrin and of the transferrin saturation.

The TIBC is the quantity of iron that can be bound by transferrin in a specified volume of serum.

The LIBC is the result obtained when the quantity of iron actually present is subtracted from the TIBC. It represents transferrin without iron.

The following relation exists:

$$TIBC = LIBC + Plasma\ Iron$$

The TIBC is measured in the routine laboratory according to Ramsay, and is performed in parallel with the determination of iron: An excess of Fe^{3+} ions is added to the serum to saturate the transferrin. The unbound Fe^{3+} ions are then precipitated with basic magnesium carbonate. After centrifugation, the iron in the clear supernatant is measured.

Iron-Binding Proteins in Serum/Plasma

All methods for the determination of plasma proteins such as ferritin and transferrin are based on the immunological principle of the reaction between an antigen (AG) and an antibody (AB). Following the addition of a suitable antiserum, this reaction leads to the formation of an immune complex of the antigen (the protein to be determined) and the antibody:

$$AG + AB = AGAB$$

$$AG = antigen, AB = antibody, AGAB = immunocomplex$$

The antibodies used must have a high specificity as well as high affinity for the antigen.

A distinction is made between polyclonal antibodies, which are mixtures from different cell lines, and monoclonal antibodies, which are derived from a single cell line. The latter are produced by the procedure published by Köhler and Milstein [102], and are identical in their antigen specificity and in their antigen-binding behavior.

The initially formed antigen-antibody complex cannot be observed directly if the antigen concentration is very low. In this case either the

Laboratory

antigen or the antibody must be labeled in order to make a measurement possible. The label may be e.g. an enzyme, a radioactive isotope, or a fluorescent dye. These indirect methods are particularly suitable for the determination of very low antigen concentrations, as in the case of ferritin.

With higher antigen concentrations, the initial reaction between the antigen and the antibody may be followed by agglutination or precipitation as a secondary reaction. The results can then be measured directly, and are often visible. The direct methods are particularly suitable for determination of higher antigen concentrations, as e.g. in the case of transferrin.

The immunochemical methods used for the determination of analytes in routine laboratory work can be divided into indirect methods with labeling and direct methods [111].

The use of labels enables the automated measurement of the primary immunoreaction.

The radioimmunoassay was introduced in 1958 by Berson and Yalow. Enzyme immunoassays, fluorescence immunoassays [82], and luminescence immunoassays followed later as logical developments designed to avoid the disadvantages associated with the use of radioactive materials.

The quantitative determination of all direct immunoassays is based on the Heidelberger-Kendall curve [74], which describes the relationship between the antigen concentration and the quantity of precipitate for a constant quantity of antibody. The quantity of precipitate is measured (Fig. 53).

The ratio of the antigen concentration to the antibody concentration is particularly important in the direct methods, since this ratio directly influences the formation of the precipitate.

Table 46: Indirect measurement of the primary immuno-reaction after labeling

Marker	Assay
Enzymes	Enzyme immunoassay (EIA)
Radioactive isotope	Radioimmunoassay (RIA)
Fluorescent dye	Fluorescence immunoassay (FIA)
Luminescence-producing substances	Luminescence immunoassay (LIA)

Laboratory

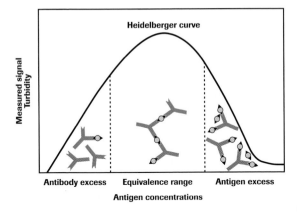

Fig. 53: Heidelberg-Kendall curve

As can be seen from the course of the Heidelberger curve, two different antigen concentrations can give the same measurement signal. This can lead to incorrect results. Quantitative immunoassays must therefore be performed below the equivalence point. The conventional method of deciding whether a signal lies on the ascending (antibody excess) or descending (antigen excess) part of the Heidelberger curve is to repeat the determination with a higher dilution of the sample. Another possibility is to add antigen or antiserum to the reaction mixture. Modern automated analyzers can virtually eliminate this source of error by means of check functions (characterization and automatic redilution of the sample). Most manufacturers of immunochemical reagents declare the concentration range in which no antigen excess problem arises, i.e., no high-dose hook effect is found.

Table 47: Direct measurement methods

Marker	Assay
Measurement of the precipitate in solution	Turbidimetric immunoassay
	Nephelometric immunoassay
Measurement of the agglutination of coated particles	Latex immunagglutination assays
Precipitate in gels	Radial immunodiffusion

Ferritin

The ferritin that can be detected in the blood is in equilibrium with the body's storage iron, and can thus serve as an index [95, 114] of the size of the iron stores.

Ferritin is not a uniform molecule. It occurs in different tissues as various isoferritins. These isoferritins are constructed from two subunits, the H-(heavy)-type subunit and the L-(light)-type subunit (Fig. 54).

For the clinical evaluation of the body's iron stores by determination of the ferritin, the ferritin antibodies must possess specificity for the basic L-rich isoferritins from iron storage tissues (marrow, liver, spleen), whereas their reactivity with acidic H-rich isoferritins (e.g. from cardiac muscle) should be as low as possible.

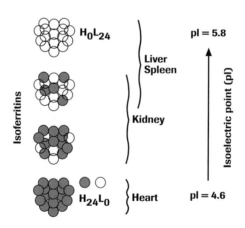

Fig. 54: Organ-specific isoferritins

Among the label-free immunoassay methods, latex-enhanced agglutination tests are particularly suitable for detection of the very low plasma ferritin concentration. Among the immunoassay methods with labels, enzyme immunoassays (EIAs), LIAs, FIAs, and RIAs are widely used.

Ferritin in plasma/serum must be determined in a very low concentration range ($0.2-7 \times 1012$ mol/L). A sufficiently sensitive method is therefore essential. In recent years, the sensitivity of the direct methods (turbidimetry, nephelometry) has been improved considerably.

Parallel to the development of the methods, success was also achieved in effort to automate the various direct and indirect immunochemical methods.

There is (at present) no reference method for the determination of ferritin.

International efforts towards a uniform standardization of ferritin are being coordinated by the WHO (World Health Organization), the ICSH (International Committee of Standardization in Hematology), the IFCC (International Federation of Clinical Chemistry), and the IUIS (Standardization Committee of the International Union of Immunological Societies).

Table 48: Historical survey

Year	Milestone
1972	Development of an immunoradiometric assay (IRMA) (Addison et al.)
1984	Turbidimetric test with reaction enhancement by latex (Bernard et al.)
1984	ICHS ferritin standard defined
1997	3rd International Standard, Recombinant

Table 49: Ferritin methods

Radioimmunoassay (RIA)
Turbidimetric latex agglutination test
Enzyme-linked immunosorbent assay (ELISA)
Nephelometric immunoassay
Fluorescence immunoassay (FIA)
Luminescence immunoassay (LIA)

Ferritin is a mixture of various isoferritins. The prerequisite for uniform standardization is a defined ferritin preparation with a high content of basic isoferritins. The ICHS (Expert Panel of Iron) has had a defined ferritin standard (human liver ferritin) since 1984. Since 1997

Laboratory

theWHO 3ʳᵈ International Standard for Ferritin, recombinant (94/572) has been available [185].

Many of the modern commercially available ferritin methods exhibit good specificity, precision, and sensitivity within their field of application and show good agreement in comparisons with one another (Fig. 55).

Ferritin, like transferrin, but unlike iron, shows no appreciable circadian rhythm. In view of the effect of an upright body position on high molecular weight blood components, the blood collection conditions must be standardized with regard to body position and venous occlusion.

Preferably the same sample should be used for the ferritin determinations as for the iron, transferrin and soluble transferrin receptor (sTfR).

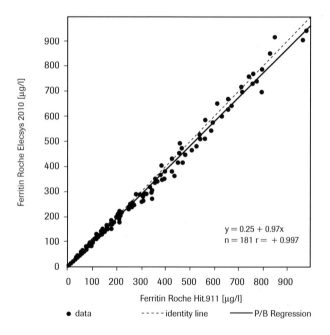

$$y = 0.25 + 0.97x$$
$$n = 181 \quad r = +0.997$$

● data   - - - - identity line   —— P/B Regression

Fig. 55: Comparison of turbidimetric and ELISA methods for the determination of ferritin

Reference Range:

The determination of reference ranges for the ferritin concentrations of clinically healthy individuals is extremely difficult, since iron stores are strongly dependent on age and sex (Fig. 56), and a significant fraction of the "normal population" suffers from latent iron deficiency. This limits the usefulness of selected reference groups, such as regular blood donors, or individuals subject to military service, or even young female hospital staff. The reference values listed have been compiled from several studies with well-defined "normal study populations". In particular, individuals with iron deficiency anemia (manifest iron deficiency) and infections (clinical examination, laboratory results) were excluded.

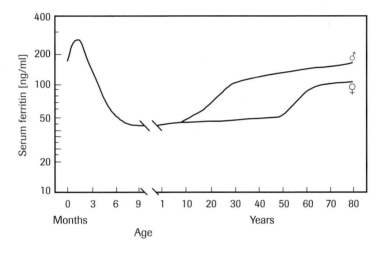

Fig. 56: Age and sex dependence of the serum ferritin concentration

Reference range:

Ferritin concentrations in healthy individuals: Lotz, J et al (1999) Clin Chem Lab med 37 (8) 821-825

Children and adolescents (4 months to 16 years)	15-150 ng/mL
Men	30-400 ng/mL
Women under 50 years of age	15-150 ng/mL
Women over 50 years of age	Approximation to the reference interval for men

Remark:

• Babies initially have full iron stores, which are used up within a few weeks.

• The indicated reference ranges statistically cover 95% of clinically healthy population groups. They do not by any means represent an ideal norm.

Transferrin (Tf)

Half of the body's transferrin is contained in the serum/plasma, while the other half is extravascular. The protein is able to transport two tri-valent iron ions per molecule. 30 to 40% of this maximum binding capacity is utilized under physiological conditions.

Transferrin is not a uniform molecule. It is a group of various iso-transferrins. Presently approximately 20 human isotransferrins are known. They all have the same iron-binding capacity and similar immunological characteristics. Therefore distinguishing between the various isoforms has no practical value for the assessment of iron metabolism. Since the technical requirements for the determination of transferrin in the routine laboratory are relatively simple, the determination of the transferrin in serum/plasma has displaced the determination of the TIBC (total iron-binding capacity) and of the LIBC (latent iron-binding capacity).

Table 50: Historical survey

Year	Milestones
1958	Determination of transferrin by radial immunodiffusion, RID (Ramsey)
1976	Turbidimetric determination of transferrin (Kreutzer)
1978	Nephelometric determination (Buffone)

Methods:

There is (at present) no reference method for the determination of transferrin. Because of the relatively high transferrin concentration (25-45 mmol/L), direct immunological precipitation methods (nephelometry, turbidimetry) are suitable. Turbidimetric and nephelometric methods are widely used as routine methods.

Transferrin, like ferritin, but unlike iron, shows no pronounced circadian rhythm. In view of the effect of an upright body position on high molecular weight blood components, the blood collection conditions for transferrin determinations must again be standardized with regard to body position and vein constriction. Preferably the same sample should be used for the transferrin determination as for iron and ferritin.

Reference range for transferrin:

No major dependence on age or sex is found [75].

200-400 [mg/dL]	25-50 [μMol/l]

Relationship between Transferrin and Total Iron Binding Capacity (TIBC)

Table 51: Relationship between transferrin and TIBC

Relationship between Transferrin and TIBC	Reference ranges
Transferrin [μmol/L] x 2 ~ TIBC [μmol/L]	Transferrin: 25 - 50 [μmol/L] w: TEBK: 49 – 89 [μmol/L] m: TEBK: 52 - 77 [μmol/L]
Transferrin [mg/dL] x $\frac{2 \times 56}{79\,570}$ ~ TIBC [μg/dL]	Transferrin: 200 - 400 [mg/dL] w: TEBK: 274 – 497 [μg/dL] m: TEBK: 291 – 430 [μg/dL]
Transferrin [mg/dL] x 1.41 ~ TIBC [μg/dL]	

The following has been taken into account:

• 1 mol of transferrin binds 2 atoms of iron

• Atomic weight of iron = 56 daltons

• Molecular weight of APO transferrin = 79,570 daltons [72]

Remark:
Total Iron Binding Capacity (TIBC) of 1 g transferrin is 1.41 mg iron.

Transferrin Saturation (TfS)

Transferrin saturation is defined as the ratio of the serum/plasma iron concentration to the serum/plasma transferrin concentration (multiplied by a correction factor). It is a dimensionless quantity, so that unlike iron, it is independent of the patient's state of hydration:

$$\text{Transferrin saturation in \%} = \frac{\text{iron } [\mu mol/L] \text{ x } 100}{\text{transferrin } [\mu mol/L]}$$

$$= \frac{\text{iron } [\mu g/dL] \text{ x } 100 \text{ x } 56}{\text{transferrin } [\mu g/dL] \text{ x } 79\,570}$$

$$= \frac{\text{iron } [\mu g/dL] \text{ x } 100 \text{ x } 56 \text{ x } 1\,000}{\text{transferrin } [mg/dL] \text{ x } 79\,570}$$

$$= \frac{\text{iron } [\mu g/dL] \text{ x } 100}{\text{transferrin } [mg/dL] \text{ x } 1.41}$$

56 = Atomic weight of iron in daltons
79 570 = Molecular weight of APO transferrin in daltons [72]

Reference range:
Transferrin saturation [75]

Transferrin saturation in healthy individuals	15 - 45 %
Decreased transferrin saturation in iron deficiency or disturbances of iron distribution	< 15 %
Elevated transferrin saturation in iron overload	> 50 %

Remarks:
- *Transferrin saturation of 10 % expresses that 1 g transferrin is saturated with 0.141 mg iron.*
- *Transferrin saturation of 50 % is reached, when 1 g transferrin contains 0.705 mg iron.*

Laboratory

Soluble Transferrin Receptor (sTfR)

The membrane-bound transferrin receptor is a glycoprotein and is made of two identical chains bound via disulfide bonds with a molecular weight of 95,000 daltons each. The transferrin receptor is a transmembrane protein of many cells of the body. It binds iron-loaded transferrin to the cell surface and transports it inside the cell.

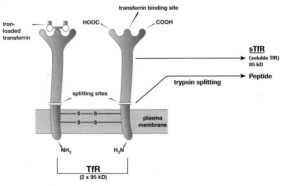

Fig. 57: Transferrin receptor (TfR)

The soluble serum transferrin receptor (sTfR) released into the blood is a monomer of approximately 85,000 daltons. It is produced after the proteolytic splitting of approximately 100 amino acids from the bound transferrin receptor [35, 36, 87].

There is still no reference method for determining the soluble serum transferrin receptor.

On account of the relatively low concentration of soluble serum transferrin receptor in the blood (< 10 mg/L or < 100 nmol/L), only sufficiently sensitive measuring methods are suitable for the determination.

Enzyme immunoassays, radio immunoassays, and latex-enhanced immunonephelometric methods are the methods most frequently used for routine determinations. A recommended standard is not yet available. To calibrate the assays, human sera-based preparations of intact TfR, the complex of TfR with transferrin or mixtures are used. This results in values that cannot be compared between the various assays.

In the latex-enhanced immunoassay, the sTfR molecule from the serum sample reacts with the anti-sTfR-antibody (monoclonal, mouse) and forms an antigen/antibody complex which is then measured turbidimetrically (Fig. 58).

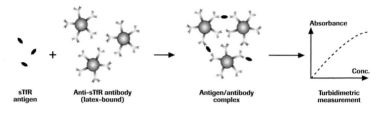

Fig. 58: Test principle of particle-enhanced immunoturbidimetric assay of soluble transferrin receptor (s-TfR)

Reference range:
Concentrations of soluble TfR (sTfR) in the serum of healthy individuals [75, 103]

Women:	(premenopausal)	1,9 – 4,4 mg/L
Men:		2,2 – 5,0 mg/L

There is a good direct proportional relationship between

• The expression of the amount of TfR on the erythrocytes and the concentration of sTfR,
• and the mass of erythropoietic cells and the concentration of sTfR in the plasma.

The concentration of sTfR is therefore raised in the presence of increased expression of TfR, as is the case with active iron deficiency, and in hyperproliferative erythropoiesis. These states can be differentiated by performing an additional determination of ferritin and the reticulocyte count.

Haptoglobin

The haptoglobin detectable in the serum binds the hemoglobin resulting from pathologically increased hemolysis in a fixed haptoglobin-hemoglobin (Hp-Hb) complex. A decrease in the free haptoglobin thus serves as an indicator of intravascular hemolysis.

The 1:1 Hp-Hb complex is incorporated into the hepatocytes with a half-life of less than 10 min. There, the hemoglobin is enzymatically metabolized. The haptoglobin released is returned to the serum with a half-life of about 3 days.

The formation of the fixed Hp-Hb complex and its extremely rapid elimination from the bloodstream prevents hemoglobinuria with severe renal iron loss.

Haptoglobin is a glycoprotein structurally related to the immuno-globulins, and is made up of 2 light (α) chains with a molecular weight of 9000 daltons and two heavier (β) chains (molecular weight: 16,000 daltons). Three phenotypes with different molecular weights are known: Hp 1-1, Hp 2-1 and Hp 2-2. Hp 1-1 has a molecular weight of 100,000 daltons. Hp 2-1 and Hp 2-2 are high-molecular-weight polymers with a molecular weight ranging from 200,000 to 400,000 daltons.

Methods:

There is (at present) no reference method for the determination of haptoglobin. Because of the relatively high haptoglobin concentration in the serum (30 - 200 mg/dL), direct immunological precipitation methods (e.g., nephelometry, turbidimetry) are suitable. Turbidimetric and nephelometric methods are widely used as routine methods.

Table 52: Historical survey

Year	Milestones
1960	Haptoglobin-hemoglobin binding test; determination of free haptoglobin in serum (Nyman)
1987	Turbidimetric test for haptoglobin (Johnson)

Reference range:

Haptoglobin concentrations in the serum of healthy persons. There are no major differences based on age or sex [75].

Adults	30 - 200 mg/dL	0.3 – 2.0 g/L

CRM 470 standardized

Laboratory

Remarks:

• Neonates have no measurable haptoglobin levels in the first 3 months; the reference range for adults applies from the 4th month.

• The reference range is dependent on the phenotype:

		[mg/dL]	[g/L]
Hp 1 - 1	w:	91 – 160	0.91 – 1.60
	m:	87 – 142	0.87 – 1.42
Hp 2 - 1	w:	82 – 124	0.82 – 1.24
	m:	74 – 124	0.74 – 1.24
Hp 2 – 2	w:	58 – 99	0.58 – 0.99
	m:	52 – 101	0.52 – 1.01

Like ferritin and transferrin haptoglobin shows no appreciable circadian rhythm. In view of the effect of an upright body position on high molecular weight blood components, the blood collection conditions must be standardized with regard to body position and venous occlusion. The haptoglobin determination should preferably be performed using the same serum sample as for the other iron metabolism parameters.

In presence of massive hemolysis - when no haptoglobin concentration is detectable - hemopexin (Hpx) should be measured [135].

Ceruloplasmin (Cp)

Ceruloplasmin is α-glycoprotein with a molecular mass of 132 kDa and contains about 9% carbohydrate. The Cp molecule binds 6-8 Cu atoms.

Cp is synthesized mostly in the liver. Its functions include:
• transport of copper (Cu) in plasma
• ferroxidase activity; it oxidizes Fe^{2+} to Fe^{3+}

New insights have been gained concerning the role of ceruloplasmin in iron metabolism. The "endo-oxidase activity" of this copper transporting protein seems to be important for intracellular oxidation of Fe^{2+} to Fe^{3+} which is necessary for release of iron ions from the cells and the binding to transferrin. This is exemplified by the very rare hereditary aceruloplasminemia where the lack of iron oxidation prevents binding to transferrin and thereby leads to intracellular trapping of iron ions and consequently to the development of an iron overload which resembles hereditary hemochromatosis. However, in contrast to hemochromatosis the central nervous system is also affected. Due to the impaired transferrin binding, however, iron concentrations and transferrin saturation in plasma are low whereas ferritin concentrations are high, reflecting the impaired iron distribution and release. In this case, therefore, disturbance of iron distribution occurs in addition to the iron overload.

• Antioxidative effect, due to the prevention of metal ion-catalyzed oxidation of lipids in the cell membrane
• acute phase protein in inflammation.

Methods of determination:
Ceruloplasmin antibodies react with the antigen from the sample with formation of an antigen-antibody complex which is measured after agglutination using turbidimetry.

Reference range:
Ceruloplasmin concentrations in the serum of healthy persons. There are no major differences based on age or sex [75].

Adults	15 - 60 mg/dL	0.15 – 0.6 g/L

Determination of Vitamin B_{12} and Folic Acid

The diagnostic value of determining vitamin B_{12} and folic acid - mainly in macrocytic anemic states - is beyond dispute. All modern vitamin B_{12} and folate determinations in serum are based on an immunological analysis method. Because the indication is the same in virtually all cases, it is customary and often useful to determine folic acid and vitamin B_{12} in the plasma simultaneously as a double assay.

Laboratory

Vitamin B$_{12}$

Vitamin B$_{12}$ has a molecular weight of 1355 daltons and, as cyanocobalamin, belongs to a biologically active substance group which has as common structural element a porphyrin ring with cobalt as the central atom.

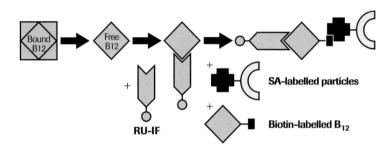

SA-labelled particles

RU-IF

Biotin-labelled B$_{12}$

Step 1:
Denaturation
of sample
and release
of B$_{12}$

Step 2:
Addition of
ruthenium
(RU)-labelled
intrinsic factor (IF)
and coupling
to B$_{12}$
→ RU-IF-B$_{12}$

Step 3:
Addition of streptavidin (SA)-
loaded particles (beads) and
competitive reaction of biotin-
labelled B$_{12}$ with endogenous B$_{12}$

Fig. 59: Test principle of an immunochemical determination of vitamin B$_{12}$
           based on electrochemiluminescence (ECL) (according to B.C. Trauth).

The vitamin B$_{12}$ taken in with food or synthesized by intestinal bacteria ("extrinsic factor") forms a complex with the "intrinsic factor", a glycoprotein formed in the gastric mucosa. Formation of this complex serves to protect the vitamin from degradation in the intestine and facilitates its receptor-dependent absorption by the mucosa of the small intestine. After dissociation of the vitamin B$_{12}$ "intrinsic factor", complex the vitamin can be transported to the liver, where it is stored. In the cells, the vitamin is present mainly as 5′-deoxyadenosyl-cobalamin, whereas methylcobalamin predominates in the plasma. Transcobalamin II (TC-II) serves as the most important transport protein for vitamin B_{12} in the plasma.

Table 53: Historical survey

Year	Milestones
1950	Microbiological determination of Lactobacillus leichmannii (Mathews)
1962	Radioimmunological determination (Bavakat, Ekins)
1978	Use of highly purified intrinsic factor as binding protein (Kolhouse)
1986	Automated determination of B_{12}/folate (Henderson)

A microbiological assay is recommended by the NCCLS as reference method for the research laboratory. The biological activity of vitamin B_{12} is measured in relation to the growth of the microorganisms E. gracilis or L. leichmannii. It is not suitable for wider use because of the apparatus required and the specificity of the technique.

A considerable advance in methods was made in 1962 with the introduction of a radioimmunoassay. The determination is based on the competitive binding of radiolabeled vitamin B_{12} and the free vitamin B_{12} in the sample to the intrinsic factor. Before the determination is performed, vitamin B_{12} is released from the endogenous binding proteins in a thermal stage or by pretreatment in an alkaline solution.

False normal results that led to the non-detection of a vitamin B_{12} deficiency were corrected using highly purified intrinsic factor free of (rapidly migrating) R proteins. The method described in Kolhouse in 1978 makes it possible to exclude binding of endogenous cobalamin analogs in the serum to nonspecific R proteins in the immunological test.

Vitamin B_{12} in the serum or plasma must be determined in a very low concentration range (50-1500 pg/ml). This calls for a sufficiently sensitive method. The list of milestones shows that the first generation of determination methods was based exclusively on indirect measure-

Laboratory

ment by radioimmunoassay. In 1986 Henderson, Friedman et al. introduced a non-radioactive immunoassay. This elegant measurement principle made it possible to substantially increase the sensitivity of the direct-measurement method and apply a homogeneous immunoassay for vitamin B_{12} on existing routine analyzers without first performing a thermal stage.

Reference range:

Vitamin B_{12} concentrations in the serum of healthy persons. There are no major differences based on age or sex [75].

Adults	220 - 925 pg/mL	162 - 683 pmol/L

Remarks:

• Given a daily requirement of 30 µg/d vitamin B_{12}, parental administration of vitamin B_{12} often leads to raised concentrations after a few months. The vitamin B_{12} pool is approximately 3 – 7 mg.
• In about 20% of pregnant women, the vitamin B_{12} concentration in the serum falls to values of < 125 pmol/l despite adequate depots.
• Some of the reference ranges for vitamin B_{12} given in the literature differ considerably. This is undoubtedly due to the considerable differences in methods used in the past.
• Findings from Brouwer [24] and Herrmann [81] suggest that the reference ranges for folic acid and vitamin B_{12} should be increased.

Folic Acid

Folic acid is a pteridine derivative and is present as a conjugate with several glutaminic acid molecules. After the ingestion of food it is initially hydrolyzed enzymatically to pteroylmonoglutaminic acid (PGA) in the mucosal epithelium of the small intestine. Reduction and methylation then take place in the intestinal wall; the resultant N-5-methyl-tetrahydrofolic acid (MTHFA) is released into the bloodstream. Tetrahydrofolic acid (THFA) is formed from MTHFA under the influence of vitamin B_{12}. It is involved in numerous reactions as a coenzyme.

The microbiological assay recommended as reference method is unsuitable for widespread use. Measurements are made of the biological activity of N-5-methyltetrahydrofolic acid (MTHFA) in relation to the growth of Lactobacillus casei.

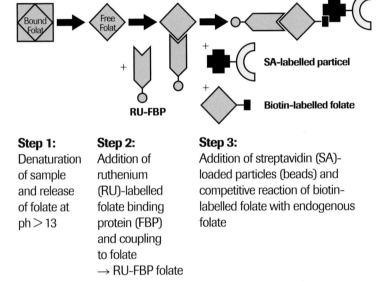

Step 1:
Denaturation of sample and release of folate at ph > 13

Step 2:
Addition of ruthenium (RU)-labelled folate binding protein (FBP) and coupling to folate
→ RU-FBP folate

Step 3:
Addition of streptavidin (SA)-loaded particles (beads) and competitive reaction of biotin-labelled folate with endogenous folate

Fig. 60: Test principle of an immunochemical determination of folate based on electrochemiluminescence (ECL) (according to B. C. Trauth).

A major advance in methods was achieved in 1973 with the introduction of the radioimmunological competitive protein binding test. The determination is based on the competitive binding of radiolabeled N-5-methyltetrahydrofolic acid (MTHFA) (125J-MTHFA) and the N-5-methyltetrahydrofolic acid (MTHFA) of the sample to the binding protein β-lactoglobulin. Before the determination is performed, MTHFA is released from the endogenous binding proteins in a thermal stage or by pretreatment in an alkaline solution. The false normal results observed in individual cases which, compared with the microbiological reference method, failed to reveal a folic acid deficiency, can be corrected by using a chromatographically highly purified β-lactoglobulin free from non-specific binding proteins.

Laboratory

Table 54: Historical survey

Year	Milestones
1966	Microbiological determination of N-5-methyl-tetrahydrofolic acid (MTHFA) with Lactobacillus casei (Herbert)
1973	Determination of folic acid by radioimmunoassay (Dunn)
1978	Use of highly purified β-lactoglobulin (Kohlhouse)
1986	Automated determination of B_{12}/folate (Henderson)

Folic acid in the serum or plasma must be determined in a very low concentration range (0.5-20 ng/mL). This calls for a sufficiently sensitive method. The list of milestones shows that the first generation of determination methods was based exclusively on indirect measurement with a radioimmunoassay. Immunoassays have recently become commercially available which do not use radioisotopes but employ an elegant, simple reaction for separating folic acid from the endogenous binding proteins. In 1986 Henderson introduced an immunological folate determination using the direct-measurement method for use on existing routine analyzers without first performing a thermal stage (Fig. 60).

Remarks:
• Because of the close connection between vitamin B_{12} and folic acid in the metabolism and the difficulty of hematological and clinical differentiation between the two vitamin deficiency states, it is advisable to determine both parameters simultaneously in patients with the relevant vitamin deficiency symptoms.

Reference ranges:
Folic acid concentrations in the serum of healthy persons. There are no major differences based on age or sex [75].

Adults	2.7 – 16.1 ng/mL	6.1 – 36.5 nmol/L

• Given a daily requirement of approximately 200 μg/d and a total content in the body of about 5-10 mg, parental administration of folic acid (e.g., in absorption tests) often leads to raised concentrations of folic acid after a few weeks.

- Some of the reference ranges for folic acid given in the literature differ considerably. This is undoubtedly due to the considerable differences in methods used in the past.
- Findings from Brouwer [24] and Herrmann [81] suggest that the reference ranges for folic acid and vitamin B_{12} should be increased.

Erythropoietin

Table 55: Properties of Erythropoietin

Molecular Properties	EPO is an acidic glycoprotein
	• The non-processed protein consists of 193 amino acids. To form the "mature" EPO polypeptide, a 27-amino acid-fragment is split from the N-terminus, and a single arginine group is split from the C-terminus.
	• The processed protein consists of 165 amino acids.
Molecular weight	Depending on carbohydrate side chains, the molecular weight can fluctuate between 30,000 and 34,000.
Protein structure	• EPO contains two disulfide bonds, at least one of which is important for the biological activity of the molecule.
	• The individual polypeptide chain is responsible for stimulting the target cells.
	• The four carbohydrate side chains determine the stability and pharmacokinetic properties of the molecule (in particular the rate at which EPO is eliminated from the bloodstream).

EPO is a glycoprotein that controls a feedback mechanism to maintain a constant erythrocyte mass in the body. Increased release of EPO leads to erythrocytosis and a reduction in erythrocytopenia.

In adults, 80-90% of EPO is formed in the kidneys. Extrarenal formation sites include the liver and macrophages. The kidney is merely a synthesis organ of EPO, i.e., it is synthesized there as needed.

The focus of erythropoietin determination in clinical diagnostics lies in the differential diagnosis of erythrocytosis. The significance of the differential diagnosis of anemias is increasing. Other indications are suspicion of renal anemia and determination of the starting value before initiating treatment of anemia with recombinant human EPO.

A reference method for the determination of erythropoietin does not exist at this time. Due to the extremely low concentration of EPO in serum, methods of determination must be highly sensitive. Radio immunoassays and commercially available enzyme immunoassays are the most popular routine methods.

Sandwich Enzyme Immunoassay:

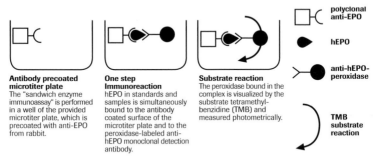

Antibody precoated microtiter plate
The "sandwich enzyme immunoassay" is performed in a well of the provided microtiter plate, which is precoated with anti-EPO from rabbit.

One step Immunoreaction
hEPO in standards and samples is simultaneously bound to the antibody coated surface of the microtiter plate and to the peroxidase-labeled anti-hEPO monoclonal detection antibody.

Substrate reaction
The peroxidase bound in the complex is visualized by the substrate tetramethyl-benzidine (TMB) and measured photometrically.

polyclonal anti-EPO

hEPO

anti-hEPO-peroxidase

TMB substrate reaction

Fig. 61: Reaction scheme of an enzyme immunoassay

The analytical sensitivity of the enzyme immunoassay is approximately 1 IU/l.

Interpretations of the measured EPO concentration is only possible in conjunction with hemoglobin or hematocrit levels. Interpretations of EPO reference ranges alone have no clinical relevance.

Both a decrease and an increase in the production of EPO are of diagnostic significance. Both conditions can be detected by measuring serum EPO concentration.

EPO deficiency causes normocytic normochromic anemia. The most common cause is chronic renal failure because in adults EPO is almost exclusively synthesized in the kidney.

EPO overproduction occurs as a result of tissue hypoxia. In cases of non-renal anemias, EPO concentration often increases exponentially as hemoglobin concentration decreases (Fig. 62).

Reference ranges:
EPO concentrations in the serum of healthy persons. There are no major differences based on age or sex [75].

Adults	5 – 25 IU/L

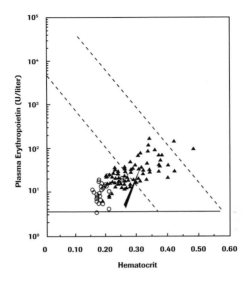

Fig. 62: Plasma erythropoietin levels in 120 patients receiving dialysis in relation to hematocrit. Open circles denote ○ anephric patients and trianles ▲ patients with kidneys. The broken lines represent ---95% confidence limits for 175 normal blood donors and patients with anemia. The solid line represents the limit of detection of the assay.
(From Ersley AJ: Erythropoietin. N Engl J Med 324: 1339-1344, 1991)

The Blood Count

The complete blood cell count of the small (red) and large (red and white) blood count is performed today using modern, fully-automated hematology analyzers. EDTA whole blood is used as the sample for the cell count. The following parameters are determined or calculated from other parameters:
• hemoglobin (Hb)
• hematocrit (HCT)
• red blood cell (RBC) count
• erythrocyte indices
  - mean cell volume of red cells (MCV)
  - mean cell hemoglobin content of red cells (MCH)

- mean cell hemoglobin concentration of red cells (MCHC)
- red cell distribution width (RDW)
- reticulocyte count
  - mean cell volume reticulocytes (MCVr)
  - mean cell hemoglobin concentration reticulocytes (CHCMr)
- hemoglobin content reticulocyte (CHr). CHr is the product of
  MCVr x CHCMr = CHr
- white blood cell (WBC) count
- differentiated count leukocytes (DCL) (the number of lymphocytes,
  monocytes, neutrophils, basophils and eosinophils)
- platelet (PLT) count
- mean platelet volume (MPV).

Reticulocytes, reticulocyte count, reticulocyte maturation indices, reticulocyte production index (RPI) are new parameters on hematology analyzers.

The parameters of the small (red) blood count shall be described below:

Table 56: Parameters determined in routine hematology

	Complete blood count (CBC)	Differential blood count
Information on number and type of blood cells	White blood cells (WBC)	3-part differential Lymphocytes Monocytes Granulocytes
	Red blood cells (RBC) Platelets (Plt)	5-part differential Lymphocytes Monocytes
		Neutrophils Basophils Eosinophils
The hemoglobin concentration as biochemical parameter	Hemoglobin (Hb)	
The volume of (red blood) cells as percentage of total blood volume	Hematocrit (Hct) (or packed cell volume, PCV)	
Different red blood cell indices to define size and Hb content of RBCs (calculated using Hb, RBC and Hct)	Mean cell volume (MCV) Mean cell Hb (MCH) Mean cell Hb-concentration (MCHC)	
CBC: Complete Blood Count; WBC: White Blood Cell Count; PLC: Platelet Count; RBC: Red Blood Cell Count; MCV: Mean Cell Volume; MCH: Mean Cell Hb; MCHC: Mean Cell Hb-Concentration; PVC: Packed Cell Volume		

Laboratory

The Small Blood Count

Standard hematology systems use measurement technology designed to meet the requirements for testing the 8 parameters of the small blood count (RBC, Hb, HCT, MCV, MCH, MCHC, WBC, PLT). The wide variety of hematology systems offered on the market today differ according to:

- Level of automation. Systems range from semi-automated, automated, and fully-automated analyers with different methods of sample pre-treatment and sample delivery
- Standardization and quality assurance
- Number of analytical parameters

Automated Cell Counting

Automated cell counting with a hematology system using an impedance or an optical principle is now routine in many hematology laboratories. Most hematology systems use the impedance principle. In the last few years a trend towards use of optical methods (fluorescence flow cytometry) for determination of the differential blood count has been observed. This method will dominate in the future.

Flow Cytometry

Flow cytometry measures particles in aqueous suspension, particularly single cells contained in blood and in other body fluids and cell nuclei [171].

The cells are transported in a laminar fluid stream like pearls in a chain by using a special technique (hydrodynamic focusing) and become illuminated at the interrogation point by a light beam.

The light scattered at the interrogation point by the cell is evaluated at different angles thus defining different characteristics of the cells or particles involved. The scatter characteristics strongly depend on the wavelength of the light and the particle size. For example, low-angle scattered light reflects cell size, and right-angle (orthogonal or side scatter) reflects intracellular structure.

Laboratory

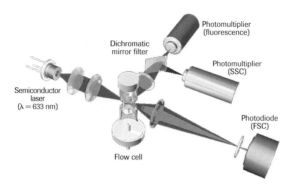

Fig. 63: Schematic illustration of a flow cytometer. New instruments offer a 3-fold combination of photomultipliers for side scatter (SSC to measure components inside the cell), forward scatter (FSC to determine cell size) and fluorescence intensity of the nucleated cells.

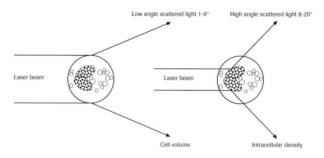

Fig. 64. Scattered light detection method

The fluorescence of cells or particles can be measured as well. Before flow cytometry cells or particles are either stained with fluorochromes or labeled with fluorescence. Excitation of fluorescence is usually by an argon laser (488 nm) emitting blue-green light or a helium-neon laser (633 nm) with red light emission. The fluorochromes therefore must have their absorption maximum near these wavelengths. Thus, depending on the application or staining technique used, either protein-fluorochrome conjugates such as fluorescent-labeled antibodies or affinity-bound dyes, e.g. thiazole orange, for reticulocyte RNA staining, are available.

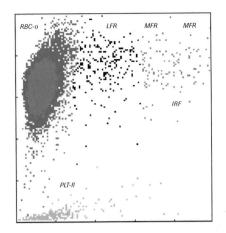

Fig. 65: Classification of reticulocytes (degree of maturity, indices)

A fluorescent dye is used for reticulocyte analysis that specifically stains the RNA and DNA of reticulate cells. More than 30,000 cells per sample are detected using flow cytometry.

Reticulocytes, erythrocytes and thrombocytes are also detected in the lowest concentration ranges.

In addition to the reticulocyte count, an additional reticulocyte differentiation is performed for a more exact assessment of bone marrow activity. When the reticulocyte matures into an erythrocyte, the DNA content of the cell decreases until the nucleic acid residue practically disappears. This biological maturation process is used for differentiation.

During the cell count in the flow cell, the fluorescence intensity as well as the intensity of the forward scatter of every single stained cell is measured. In this process, information is obtained about the nucleic acid content and size of every cell. The different degrees of maturation of the reticulocytes correspond to their fluorescence intensities. The fractions HFR (high fluorescence intensity of reticulocytes), MFR (mean fluorescence intensity of reticulocytes) and LRF (low fluorescence intensity of reticulocytes) are determined. Moreover, the population of very early reticulocytes - the immature reticulocyte fraction (IRF) - is analyzed.

The IRF value and the degrees of maturity are proven parameters for assessing the hematopoietic activity of the bone marrow. This information can be used for the diagnosis and therapy of anemias and to assess the status of the red cell line.

Typically, 5-6 parameters are measured simultaneously, e.g., cell size, intracellular density, and fluorescences of various colors.

The Impedance Principle

EDTA blood is diluted with a defined volume of electrolyte solution and placed in a transducer chamber which is connected with a further electrolyte solution via a small orifice (50-100 mm). A constant electric current is applied between electrodes on either side of the orifice. The cell suspension is drawn through the measuring orifice by means of a vacuum. When a cell passes through the orifice it acts as non-conducter and the resistance increases. Using Ohm's law, a pulse proportionate to the volume can be derived (Fig. 66). In systems using absolute measurement (number of cells per volume), the counting volume is determined with the help of manometers. Systems using the principle of relative measurement determine the cell count per unit of time. In this case the counting rate must them be converted to the cell count per volume with the help of a calibration solution (Fig. 67).

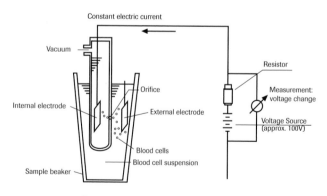

Fig. 66: Impedance principle for particle counting instrument scheme

The measuring principle for particle counting illustrated in Fig. 66 using an absolute measuring system permits the counting of red cells, white cells and platelets. On account of their different concentrations, these three parameters must be counted in two different dilutions (Fig. 67).

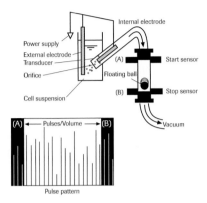

Fig. 67: Impedance principle (absolute counting) with pulse pattern; pulse counting per unit of volume

In a first dilution the white cells are analyzed after the erythrocytes have been lysed by a lysing agent. In a second, higher dilution the red cells and platelets are counted. On account of their different sizes, red cells and platelets can be differentiated from each by pulse thresholds known as discrim-inators. Many systems use variable thresholds, i.e. the ideal discriminators are determined for each sample measured. This prevents parts of a cell population from being cut off and therefore not included in the count.

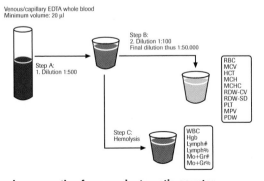

Fig. 68: Sample preparation for a semiautomatic counter

Laboratory

Hemoglobin (Hb)

The hemoglobins in the blood comprise a group of hemoglobin derivatives, namely:
• Deoxyhemoglobin (HHb)
• Oxyhemoglobin (O2Hb)
• Carboxyhemoglobin (COHb)
• Hemiglobin (Hi), also called methemoglobin (MetHb)

These hemoglobin derivatives, which are present in cell-bound form, are determined as total hemoglobin (Hb) in whole blood. Free hemoglobin, that is the hemoglobin released from the erythrocytes, however, is determined in plasma.

Measurement of Hemoglobin

Photometric measurement of hemoglobin is an integral part of present-day hematology systems. The measurement is performed either with part of the leukocyte dilution, in which case the hemoglobin released by lysis of the red cells is transformed into stable derivatives and measured photometrically, or in a separate dilution with a lysing agent specially designed for hemoglobin determination. The latter procedure has the advantage that the lysing agent used is optimized for hemoglobin measurement. There is therefore no need to take into account the sensitivity of the leukocytes and the dilution ration most appropriate for hemoglobin determination can be used. A separate hemoglobin channel with a separate hemoglobin lysing agent is subject to less interference by high leukocyte concentrations than hemoglobin photometry as part of the WBC counting.

In the past many hematology systems used a modified cyanmethemoglobin method for hemoglobin determination. This has the disadvantage that the solution contains cyanide and must therefore be disposed of as toxic waste. The introduction of a cyanide-free hemoglobin reagent has largely eliminated this problem. This reagent contains sodium lauryl sulfate as active component.

Principle of the Hemiglobincyanide Method

In solution, the Fe^{2+} of hemoglobin is oxidized to Fe^{3+} by potassium ferricyanide [$K_3Fe(CN)_6$] forming hemiglobin (Hi). This reacts with the cyanide ions (CN⁻) made available in the solution by potassium cyanide, forming cyanmethemoglobin (HiCN). The absorbance of HiCN is measured at 540 nm. The hemiglobincyanide method is the reference method [126].

$$Hb(Fe^{2+}) \xrightarrow{K_3Fe(CN)_6} \text{Methemoglobin } (Fe^{3+}) \xrightarrow{KCN} \text{Cyanmethemoglobin (HiCN)}$$

Reference range:
Hemoglobin concentrations in the serum of healthy persons [75]

Women:	12.3 – 15.3 g/dL	7.6 – 9.5 mmol/l
Men:	14.0 – 17.5 g/dL	8.7 – 10.9 mmol/l

Hematocrit (Hct)

The hematocrit, or packed cell volume (PCV), is the ratio of the volume of red cells to the volume of whole blood in a sample of venous or capillary blood. The ratio is measured after appropriate centrifugation. In laboratory practice the hematocrit is usually expressed as a percentage.

$$Hct\ (\%) = \frac{Volume_{\text{ of Erythrocytes}}}{Volume_{\text{ of whole blood}}} \times 100$$

The hematocrit is a further important parameter in laboratory hematology. This value is also determined automatically by many hematology systems today. Figure 69 shows a schematic comparison of pulse height summation, the method used by many hematology systems, and the centrifugal hematocrit. The cells which pass through the measuring orifice generate pulses which are proportionate to their volume. The hematocrit is obtained by summation of the individual pulses which are between an upper and lower discriminator. The result is multiplied by a constant factor which takes into account the dilution ratio. The hematocrit represents the percentage by volume of erythrocytes to the total volume of the blood sample. The results of the hematology analyzers are standardized against the microhematocrit method.

Laboratory

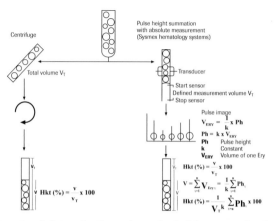

Fig. 69: Hematocrit determination using pulse height summation in comparison with centrifugation.

Microhematocrit method:

Borosilicate or soda-lime glass capillary tubes having a length of 75 mm and an internal diameter of 1.15 mm are recommended. The wall thickness should be 0.20 mm. The requirements for centrifugation are as follows:

• Microhematocrit centrifuge with a rotor radius > 8 cm
• Maximum speed should be reached within 30 sec
• Relative centrifugal force 10,000 - 15,000 x g at the periphery for 5 min without exceeding a temperature of 45° C.

The hematocrit is calculated as follows:

$$\text{Hct} = \frac{\text{Length of red cell column (mm)}}{\text{Length of red cell column plus plasma column (mm)}}$$

The microhematocrit method is the reference method [181].

Reference range:
Hematocrit (Hct) in the serum of healthy persons [75]

Women:	35 – 47 %	0.35 – 0.47
Men:	40 – 52 %	0.40 – 0.52

Laboratory

Erythrocytes

The differentiation of stem cells to erythrocytes begins at the level of the hematopoietic stem cell (CFU-GEMM). From this stage on, all successor cells of erythropoiesis have lost their ability to renew erythropoiesis.

The hematopoietic stem cell (CFU-GEMM) differentiates into the burst forming unit erythroid (BFU-E). This stage is followed by the colony forming unit erythroid (CFU-E). After various divisions, which take several days in vivo, the cells go through a process of typical morphological and functional differentiation in the process of which they lose their proliferative capacity step by step (Fig. 70).

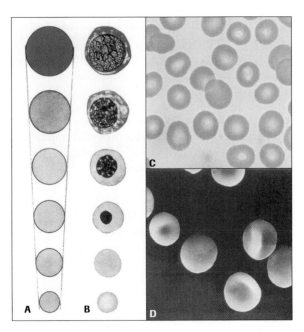

Fig. 70: A: Cell growth of erythrocytes. Cell size and color change depending
             on degree of maturity [28]
         B: Red blood cells lose nucleic acids as maturation progresses. The
             erythrocyte has virtually no nucleic acids.
         C: Erythrocytes as viewed under the microscope.
         D: Erythrocytes as viewed under the electron microscope.

As the erythrocytes age, they decrease in volume and deformability and their density increases. Changes in the cell membrane lead to loss of carbohydrates on the cell surface. The normal red cell is removed from the blood stream by the reticuloendothelial system by phagocytosis after 100-120 days.

Red Cell Count (RBC)

The red cell count is a basic examination for the evaluation of disorders of erythropoiesis.

Reference range:
Erythrocytes in the serum of healthy persons [75]

Women:	4.1 – 5.1 mil/µL
Men	4.5 – 5.9 mil/µL

Values in 10^6/µL oder 10^{12}/L

The red cell count alone is of little diagnostic value. Only the combination of this parameter with the hematocrit permits differentiation between erythrocytopenia, erythrocytosis or a normal erythrocyte count with reference to the red cell mass of the body.

RBC Indices: MCV, MCH, MCHC

Hematology analyzers calculate the following parameters from the measured red cell count and hemoglobin concentration:

• mean corpuscular volume (MCV)
• mean corpuscular hemoglobin (MCH)
• mean corpuscular hemoglobin concentration (MCHC)

The MCV, MCH and MCHC are called red cell indices and are used for the description of red cell changes and the differentiation of disturbances of erythropoiesis.

• <u>MCV = the mean cell volume of the red cell.</u>
The MCV is expressed in femtoliters (fL $\triangleq$ 10^{-15} L). Hematology analy-

zers either measure this parameter directly or calculate it according to
the following equation:

$$MCV = \frac{\text{Volume of red cells per 1}\mu\text{L blood}}{\text{Red cells per 1 }\mu\text{L blood}}$$

*The mean volume of a single erythrocyte is obtained by calculation based on
the parameters red cell concentration per microliter of blood, and hematocrit:*

$$MCV = \frac{\text{Hematocrit (Hct in \%) x 10}^{-2}}{\text{Red cell count x 10}^{6}}[\mu\text{L}] = \frac{\text{Hct in \% x 10}^{-2}\text{ x 10}^{9}}{\text{Red cell count x 10}^{6}}[\mu\text{L}]$$

$$(1 \mu\text{L} = 10^{9}\text{ fL},$$
$$(1\text{ L} = 10^{15}\text{ fL})$$

e. g.:
Red cells = 5 x 10^{6}/μL
Hematocrit = 45 %

$$MCV = \frac{45 \text{ x } 10^{-2} \text{ (x } 10^{9})}{5 \text{ x } 10^{6}} = \frac{45 \text{ x } 10}{5} = 90 \text{ fL}$$

Reference range:
MCV in the serum of healthy persons [75]

Adults	80 – 96 µm³	80 – 96 fl

Remarks:
MCV is reduced in the patients with iron deficiency, and it is raised in
patients with macrocytic anemias, reticulocytosis and aplastic anemias.

• MCH = the mean hemoglobin content of the red cell
The MCH is expressed in picograms (pg) and is obtained by calculation from the Hb concentration per microliter and the red cell count per
microliter. Hematology analyzers calculate it according to the following
equation:

$$MCH = \frac{\mu g \text{ Hb in 1 } \mu l \text{ blood}}{\text{Red cells per 1 } \mu L \text{ blood}} \text{ [pg]}$$

$$= \frac{Hb \text{ (in g/dL) x 10}}{\text{Red cells x } 10^6/\mu L} \text{ [pg]}$$

$(1 \text{ pg} = 10^{-6} \text{ } \mu g = 10^{-12} \text{ g})$

e. g.:   Red cells = 5 x 10^6/μL blood
              Hemoglobin = 16 g/dL blood = 160 g/L = 160 μg/μL

$$MCH = \frac{160 \text{ } \mu g/\mu l}{5 \text{ x } 10^6/\mu L} = 32 \text{ x } 10^{-6} \text{ } \mu g = 32 \text{ pg}$$

Reference range:

MCH in the serum of healthy persons [75]

Adult	28 – 33 pg/cell	1.7 – 2.0 fmol/cell

Remarks:

Hypochromic erythrocytes are present when MCH is less than 28 pg/cell, when Hb is more greatly reduced than red cell count, and in patients with iron deficiency or thalassemia.

Hyperchromic erythrocytes are observed when MCH is over 33 pg, and when the red cell count is more greatly reduced than Hb, or in patients with hyperchromic macrocytosis (e.g., pernicious anemia).

- MCHC = the mean hemoglobin concentration of the red cells.
  The MCHC is expressed in g/dL of red blood cells and is calculated as follows:

$$MCHC = \frac{\text{Hemoglobin concentration (g/dl)}}{\text{Hematocrit (\%)}}$$

e. g.:   Hemoglobin = 15.0 g/dL blood = 150 g/L blood
              Hematocrit = 45 % = 0,45 L red cells/L blood

$$MCHC = \frac{15 \text{ x } 100}{45} = 33 \text{ g Hb/dL red cells}$$

Reference range:
MCHC in the serum of healthy persons [75]

Adults	33 – 36 g/dL	20 – 22 mmol/L

Remarks:
MCHC is decreased in patients with serious iron deficiency and para-morphias (e.g., thalassemia). MCHC is elevated in patients with spherocytosis and exsiccosis, and in the presence of macro- and microcytic anemias.

MCV, MCH, MCHC are important for the classification of anemias and the early detection of processes which can cause anemia.

Determination of the MCV is used for the diagnostically important distinction between normocytic, microcytic and macrocytic anemias. The MCV is dependent on the hydration of the red cells and on the red cell distribution width in the plasma. In the majority of the anemias the MCH correlates with the MCV. Microcytic anemias correspond to hypochromic anemias, normocytic to normochromic anemias.

Table 57: Classification of the anemias on the basis of MCV, MCH and MCHC

Red cell indices	Evaluation
MCV reduced MCH reduced MCHC normal, reduced	Most common form of anemia: microcytic anemia Iron deficiency, ACD; disturbance of iron distribution (tumor anemias); deficiency of copper or vitamin B_6; thalassemia
MCV normal MCH normal MCHC normal	Normochromic, normocytic anemia: non regenerative anemias, e.g. chronic diseases of the kidneys, endocrine disorders, maldigestion, malabsorption, malignant tumors.
MCV normal MCH elevated / normal MCHC elevated / normal	Normocytic, normo/hyperchromic anemia: hemolysis, spherocytosis (MCHC elevated)
MCV elevated MCH normal / elevated MCHC normal / decreased	Macrocytic, hyperchromic anemia: Folate or vitamin B_{12} deficiency anemia; liver cirrhosis; Alcoholism, MDS (myelodisplastic syndrome)

Laboratory

Reticulocytes

Reticulocytes are a transitional form between the nucleated erythroblast and the anucleate mature erythrocyte. The reticulocyte is a very young erythrocyte which contains precipitated nucleic acids after supravital staining. For identification as a reticulocyte the cell must contain two or more clumps or blue-stained granules which must be visible microscopically without fine-focusing of the cell.

Reticulocytes are purged from the bone marrow into the peripheral blood approximately 18 – 36 hours before their final maturation. As such, they represent a system for the detection of the real-time status of erythropoiesis. Changes in the reticulocyte concentration in the blood correlate with the release of immature precursor stages, but not with the actual formation of blood cells in the bone marrow [25].

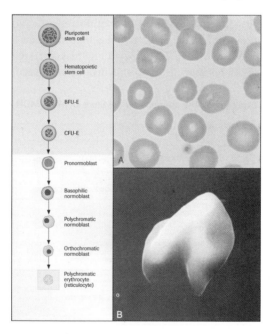

Fig. 71: Degrees of maturation of reticulocytes

    A: Polychromatic erythrocytes (reticulocytes),

    B: Electron-microscopic image of a reticulocyte according to [28]

Reticulocyte Count

Determination of the reticulocyte count is used for:

- determination of the bone marrow activity needed for renewal of RBC's consumed in the peripheral blood (e.g., suspicious of intravascular hemolysis, blood loss)
- detection of detect disturbances in RBC formation as a result of deficiencies of certain substances and monitoring the response to therapy in deficiency anemias, e.g. iron, copper, vitamin B_6, vitamin B_{12}, folate deficiency.
- evaluation of erythropoiesis after erythropoietin. In recent studies it has been proposed that response to treatment with erythropoietin be detected by measuring hemoglobin and reticulocyte count 4 weeks after starting therapy. An increase in Hb concentration by 1 g/dL or reticulocyte concentration by $> 40 \times 10^9$/L is reportedly indicative of patient response [30].
- Assessment of the marrow's ability to regenerate after cytotoxic or myeloablative therapy and bone marrow transplantation.

The reticulocyte count is expressed either as a percentage (number of reticulocytes/100 red cells) or as an absolute cell count (reticulocytes/µl).

Reference range:
Reticulocyte count in the serum of healthy persons [75]

Children (> 4 months):	$2 - 28$ ‰
	$2 - 28 \times 10^3$/µL
	$2 - 28 \times 10^9$/L
Adults	$5 - 15$ ‰
	$5 - 15 \times 10^3$/µL
	$5 - 15 \times 10^9$/L

For purposes of clinical assessment, the reticulocyte production index (RPI) should be determined as well.

The expression of reticulocytes in percent or per 100 milliliters of blood is based on mature red blood cells. The percentage can be falsely elevated when the number of mature red blood cells falls, e.g., in patients with anemia. A number of correction formula has been recommended in order to make the clinical interpretation of reticulocyte counts easier to understand:

• *Absolute reticulocyte count in blood:* reticulocyte count (per mL or per L) = % reticulocytes x RBC (per mL or per L).
 Normal value of absolute reticulocyte count: 50,000 – 100,000/μL
 The reticulocyte count expressed as per cent can be elevated either due to true replication of reticulocytes in the circulating blood or by a lower percentage of mature erythrocytes. In the case of anemia, the reticulocyte count requires a hematocrit-dependent correction expressed as the reticulocyte index.

• *Reticulocyte index:* The percentage of reticulocytes can increase due to higher reticulocyte counts or falling RBC counts. The correction can be performed based on the patient's hematocrit (Hct) with reference to an ideal Hct of 0.45:

$$\text{Reticulocyte index (RI): RI} = \text{reticulocytes (\%)} \times \frac{\text{Hct (patient)}}{0,45}$$

This correction is recommended in patients with anemias.

• Reticulocyte production index (RPI): Under normal conditions, reticulocytes become mature in the bone marrow in 3.5 days, and in 1 day while circulating in the blood.

In states of intensive erythropoietic stress, e.g., if hematocrit (Hct) drops, the maturation time of these "stress" reticulocytes in the bone marrow can be reduced to 1.5 days and, on balance, it increases in the blood. Since reticulocytes are excreted in immature stages, the number of circulating reticulocytes can increase markedly as a result without the erythropoietic activity being elevated.

The maturation time of reticulocytes in the bone marrow behaves in proportion to the Hct, i.e., it drops with Hct and, correspondingly, the maturation time in blood increases (Fig. 72). The reticulocyte count corrected for the respective maturation time and normal Hct of 0.45 is called the reticulocyte production index (RPI).

Reticulocyte production index (RPI)

$$RPI = \frac{\text{Reticulocyte count in \%}}{\text{Maturation time in blood in days}} \times \frac{\text{Hct (patient)}}{0{,}45 \text{ (ideal Hct)}}$$

Hematocrit	Dwell time of reticulocytes in blood (Shift)
45 %	1 Day
35 %	1,5 Days
25 %	2 Days
15 %	2,5 Days

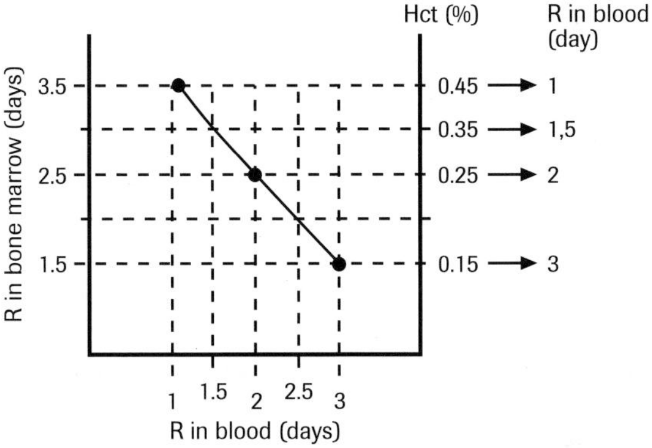

Fig. 72: Behavior of hematocrit, maturation time of reticulocytes in the bone marrow and in the peripheral blood (according to Hillmann). Hct: hematocrit

Example: Hct = 25 %, R = 20 %
          Time to maturation in blood: 2 days

$$RPI = \frac{20 \times 0.25}{2 \times 0.45}$$

In this case, erythrocyte production is increased 5.5-fold.

The reticulocyte production index is normally 1 when erythrocyte formation and degradation are in balance. In the presence of anemia, an **index value of** > 2 indicates adequate renewal. Depending on the severity of the anemia, an RPI value of < 2 indicates hypoplasia or ineffective

Laboratory

erythropoiesis. A bone marrow swab must also be obtained in order to perform a quantitative and qualitative assessment of erythropoiesis for a clinical assessment of the RPI.

In the case of normal, i.e., effective erythropoiesis, the number of reticulocytes correlates directly with renewal of red cell formation. Under an intensified effect of erythropoietin, reticulocyte maturation is shifted. The physiological time to maturation of reticulocytes is four days, three of which are spent in the bone marrow and one in the peripheral blood. The assessment of reticulocyte counts in clinical practice are based on this behavior. In the presence of anemia and depending on the hematocrit, maturation of the reticulocytes is moved to the peripheral blood with a correspondingly longer presence in the circulating blood. The changed dwell time of the reticulocytes in the peripheral blood is called the "shift". The number of reticulocytes determined in the blood must be reduced by this number in order to make a clinical statement about the actual renewal ability of erythropoiesis. Without this shift correction, the reticulocyte values determined would be too high. The real numbers are calculated in dependent on the hematocrit with the aid of the reticulocyte production index.

The maturation time to use for the Hct determined in each case is shown in Fig. 72.

The RPI can be useful in clarifying the causes of anemia. An RPI > 2.0 is associated with chronic hemolysis, bleeding or an effective therapy of existing anemia. Indices < 2.0 are associated with marrow insufficiency or ineffective erythropoiesis such as vitamin B_{12} or folic aciddeficiency anemias.

The automated reticulocyte count ensures high counting precision. In addition, the maturation index (RNA content) and the cell indices (volume, Hb content) of the reticulocytes are determined. As a result, their counting and analytical testing is gaining in clinical significance and acceptance for various diagnostic issues, especially in terms of the count results in the low range.

Hemoglobin (Hb) Content of Reticulocytes (CHr)

The mean cell volume (MCVr) of reticulocytes, the hemoglobin concentration (CHCMr), and the mathematical product of these two variables can be provided using modern hematology systems for every cell measured (MCVr-n x CHCMr-n), which corresponds to the hemoglobin content (CHr) of the reticulocytes. CHr, in particular, has proven useful in many studies in the differentiation of anemias and for monitoring erythropoietin therapy [25].

The CHr increases markedly in dialysis patients who receive i.v. iron simultaneous with EPO during therapy. This makes such a parameter an early indicator of iron-deficient erythropoiesis, even when serum ferritin or transferrin saturation are still normal [25]. In the field of pediatrics as well, CHr has proven to be a good indicator for iron deficiency in children.

Erythrocyte Ferritin

In a few studies, erythrocyte ferritin is proposed in place of serum ferritin as a parameter for anemia patients with chronic disease. The determination is not as easy to perform as for serum ferritin, and erythrocyte ferritin responds very late to dynamic changes. If, in the case of iron deficiency, practically the entire population of red blood cells has been replaced with erythrocytes having a low Hb content, erythrocyte ferritin first drops to pathologically low values. The determination of erythrocyte ferritin has not become part of daily routine testing.

Zinc Protoporphyrin

The measurement of zinc protoporphyrin (ZPP) is a rapid method, although it requires a special hematofluorimeter. Elevated ZPP values in untreated blood is very non-specific.

False positive values (pathologically raised ZPP) are observed primarily in patients with liver disease, infectious disease, and malignomas. Hastka found greatly elevated ZPP values caused by interference by various drugs [71]. Elevated values of bilirubin in the blood cause interference as well, as in the presence of cholestase, hepatitis or hemolytic anemias. ZPP contents that were apparently elevated were also found in patients with chronic kidney disease.

This apparently elevated ZPP content in the blood is caused by fluorescence interference of drugs, bilirubin or - as in the case of kidney disease - in non-dialyzable, high molecular-weight plasma components. The yellow, red or brown intrinsic colors are described as particularly disturbing [71]. On the other hand, ZPP values that are too low are measured when blood is stored. This is due to a spectral shift of deoxygenated hemoglobin.

Laboratory

Before measuring ZPP in hematofluorimeters, it is therefore recommended that the red cells be washed. This reduces ZPP normal values from 50 to 32 μmol/lmol heme. Although the ZPP determination increases in specificity as a result, the washing procedure must be performed manually. This takes a great deal of time and effort, which cancels out the advantage of the rapid automated ZPP determination.

Tests for the Diagnosis of Chronic Inflammation (ACD)

Laboratories are increasingly asked to differentiate between inflammatory and non-inflammatory diseases.
Inflammation can be detected using the following tests:

• Erythrocyte sedimentation rate (ESR)
• Quantitative determination of CRP and/or serum amyloid A protein (SAA)
• IL-6, IL-1, TNF-α determination
• Differential blood count and leukocyte count

Erythrocyte sedimentation rate (ESR)

Method of determination:
A citrated blood sample is aspirated into a glass or plastic pipette with millimeter graduation up to the 200 mm mark. The pipette remains in an upright position and the sedimentation of red cells is read off in mm after one hour. The performance of the method follows an approved guideline.

Reference range:
Erythrocyte sedimentation rate (ESR) [75]

	Less than 50 years		More than 50 years
Women	< 25 mm/1h	Women	< 30 mm/1h
Men	< 15 mm/1h	Men	< 20 mm/1h

Values in mm for the first hour.

In comparison to the quantitative determination of an acute phase protein, e.g. CRP, the ESR is also raised by an increase in the concentration of immunoglobulins, immune complexes, and other proteins. It therefore covers a broader spectrum of diseases than CRP. In the case of chronic inflammatory disease, e.g. in SLE (systemic lupus erythrematodes), in which CRP is often normal or only slightly elevated, and for monitoring in patients with these diseases, the ESR is therefore a better indicator of the inflammatory process.

C-Reactive Protein (CRP)

C-reactive protein is the classic acute phase protein that is released in response to an inflammatory reaction. It is synthesized in the liver.

CRP is composed of five identical, non-glycosylated subunits each comprising a single polypeptide chain of 206 amino acid residues with a molecular mass of 23,000 daltons. The characteristic structure places CRP in the family of pentraxins, calcium-binding proteins with immune defense properties.

CRP is synthesized rapidly in the liver following induction by IL-6. At the peak of an acute phase response, as much as 20% of the protein synthesizing capacity of the liver may be engaged in its synthesis. CRP levels increase in the plasma due to the release of inflammatory cytokines such as interleukin-6. Increased serum CRP levels are always an indicator of inflammation. However, in a malignancy such as Hodgkin's disease, the kidney cell carcinoma can also form these cytokines and prompt an acute phase response that induces fever and raised plasma concentrations of CRP.

CRP determination is used to screen for inflammatory processes [141]:
• Confirmation of the presence of acute organic disease such as cardiac infarction, deep vein thrombosis and infections; chronic conditions such as malignant tumors, rheumatic diseases, and inflammatory bowel disease. For diagnosis and monitoring of infections when microbiological testing is too slow or impossible.
• As an aid in the management of rheumatic diseases.
• For rapid establishment of the optimal anti-inflammatory therapy and the determination of the minimal effective dose.

Laboratory

Methods of determination:

Various methods of CRP determination are available, including nephelometry and turbidimetry.

CRP antibodies reagent with the antigen in the sample and form an antigen-antibody complex. This antigen-antibody complex is measured after agglutination using turbidimetry. PEG is added to reach the end point quickly, increase sensitivity, and minimize the risk of measuring false-negative levels in samples with excess antigen.

The detection sensitivity should be at least 5 mg/L and it should be lower in newborn diagnostics.

Reference range:

CRP values in adults (the values are consensus values) [75]

Adults	< 0.5 mg/dL	< 5 mg/L

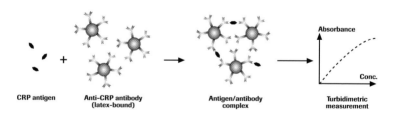

| CRP antigen | Anti-CRP antibody (latex-bound) | Antigen/antibody complex | Turbidimetric measurement |

Fig. 73: Test principle of particle-enhanced immunoturbidimetric determination of CRP (C-reactive protein)

CRP is the most sensitive of the acute phase proteins which can be readily measured in the laboratory. At present there are no clear indications for the determination of other acute phase proteins.

Although almost 30 acute phase proteins are known, only CRP and serum amyloid A (SAA) are suitable as indicators of an acute phase response. Both show a sharp increase shortly after an inflammatory stimulus and, as a result of their short half-life, a rapid drop after disappearance of the stimulus [141].

Diagnostic Significance of Cytokine Determinations

Of the many known cytokines, only the determination of a few has become established as routine diagnostic procedures, mainly IL-6, IL-1, TNF-α. They determine the extent of desired or excessive inflammatory reactions. Cytokines are not disease-specific markers.

Cytokines Regulate the Activation of the Nonspecific and Specific Immune Response

As soon as the nonspecific immune system is activated, the cytokines, TNF-α, IL-1 and IL-6 assume a central role in the induction and regulation of the nonspecific immune response. Additionally, they are a key

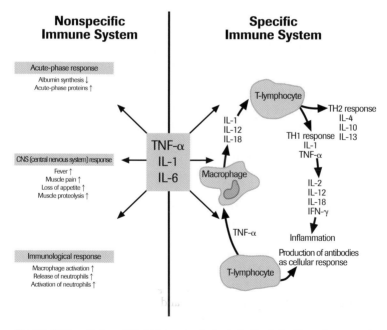

Fig. 74: TNF-α, IL-1 and IL-6 play a central role in the induction of nonspecific and specific immune responses and are decisive mediators for the differentiation of T-lymphocytes into TH1 and TH2 cells

to the specific immune response. TNF-α, IL-6 and IL-1 incite the production of many additional growth factors for the lymphocytes. IL-1 is a comitogen for T-lymphocytes. TNF-α supports the T-helper cell type 1 (TH1) T-cell response, and IL-6 is a growth factor for B-lymphocytes. This overlapping of the functions of TNF-α, IL-1 and IL-6 demonstrates the close connection between nonspecific and specific immune responses (Fig. 74). This is particularly important for the induction of nonspecific immune responses to microbiological attacks and against diseases having an autoimmune component, such as rheumatoid arthritis.

Cytokines are important in the assessment of a certain disease, since a shift in the cytokine balance can correlate with the extent of the disease-specific damage.

Tumor Necrosis Factors (TNF)

Tumor necrosis factors (TNF) are cytokines that mediate a wide range of inflammatory and immunological responses by cells to stress, infection, or injury. Two forms of homologous peptide factors are known, both of which compete for the same receptors: TNF-α, which is produced by activated monocytes and macrophages as well as by activated T-lymphocytes, and TNF-β, which is synthesized by a subpopulation of activated T-cells. The biological effects of TNF are mediated by the binding to specific receptors on the cell surfaces that are in equilibrium with the soluble TNF receptors (sTNFR).

Pathomechanisms:

An imbalanced rate of synthesis of sTNFR is found with high sTNFR levels in all infectious diseases, in acute and chronic inflammatory diseases, in injuries due to fire, sepsis, and in autoimmune diseases. Elevated concentrations are also detected in the plasma of tumor patients and subjects infected with HIV.

The tumor necrosis factor (TNF-α) plays a dominant role in the pathogenesis of numerous infectious and inflammatory diseases. TNF was named after its ability to cause hemorrhagic necrosis in tumors transplanted in laboratory animals. In 1985, TNF-α was purified and sequenced, and the gene was cloned. The main sources of TNF are monocytes and macrophages. Human TNF has a molecular weight of 26,000.

The pro-protein is split into the monomeric form by a specific metallo-proteinase (also referred to as "TNF-α-converting enzyme", TACE). The extracellular portions of both TNF-receptors are also present in the serum in soluble form. They can continue to bind TNF and thereby weaken the acute effects of the TNF.

The most sensitive method of detecting circulating TNF is based on the extremely high binding affinity and specificity of the p55-TNF receptor. No TNF was detected in the plasma of healthy subjects using this method. The detection limit of this assay is 200 attomolar (10^{-18} mol/L), corresponding to 120,000 TNF trimers or 10 femtograms in 1 ml plasma. In contrast, TNF concentrations in the nanomolar range (10^{-9} mol/L) are detected in the presence of acute diseases such as septic shock.

Interleukin-1 (IL-1)

Interleukin-1 (IL-1) is attributed with many metabolic, endocrinal, immunological, and hematological activities. Two structurally related human IL-1 molecules are known. Although IL-1 is produced by many different cell types, it is the main producing cell over the course of an antigen stimulation of the macrophage. Other IL-1-producing cells include the cells of the immune system, cells of the central nervous system, endothelial vascular cells and smooth muscle cells. IL-1 is therefore the main cause of many systemic acute-phase reactions in the case of injury and antigen-induced immune responses.

IL-1 plays an important role in the activation of the cells of the immune system. It acts on macrophages and monocytes by inducing the cytotoxic and tumor-destroying activity of these cells. It activates the B-cells to grow, differentiate, and produce immunoglobulins. IL-1 is involved in the regulation of hematopoiesis, by way of its direct effect on stem cells as well as by its ability to stimulate other cells to produce hematopoietic factors.

Pathomechanism:

An imbalanced rate of synthesis of IL-1 was found in numerous diseases. Elevated IL-1 serum levels are measured in patients with injuries, sepsis and all states of infection. IL-1 is involved in acute and chronic inflammatory diseases such as rheumatoid arthritis, inflammatory bowel disease, Alzheimer's disease, and other neurological disturbances. IL-1 contributes to the symptoms of various hematological and non-

Laboratory

hematological, malignant diseases such as multiple myeloma or acute myeloid leukemia.

Interleukin-6 (IL-6)

Interleukin-6 is synthesized by many different cell types. The main producers are stimulated monocytes, fibroblasts and endothelial cells. It is a cytokine that can trigger and inhibit cell growth. It can also trigger cell differentiation. IL-6 is reported to be an acute-phase mediator. It acts on liver cells as a hepatocyte-stimulating factor, and as a tissue hormone that induces the secretion of various acute-phase proteins such as C-reactive protein or haptoglobulin.

Pathomechanism:

An imbalanced rate of synthesis of IL-6 has been detected in the presence of numerous diseases. Elevated IL-6 levels are observed in patients with injuries due to fire, sepsis, and infection. IL-6 is involved in reactions of chronic inflammatory diseases such as rheumatoid arthritis, multiple sclerosis, Paget's bone disease and AIDS.

References

1. Aisen P (1998) Transferrin, the transferrin receptor, and the uptake of iron by cells. In: Siegel S, Siegel H. (eds). Metal ions in biological systems; Vol 35. Marcel Dekker Inc, New York: 585-631.

2. Albertini A, Arosio P, Chiancone E, Drysdale J (eds) (1984) Ferritins and isoferritins as biochemical markers. Elsevier, Amsterdam New York Oxford

3. Alford CE, King TTE, Campell PA (1991) Role of transferrin, transferrin receptors and iron in macrophage listericidal activity. J Med 174; 45: 9-466

4. Andrews NC (1999) Disorders of iron metabolism. N Engl J Med 341: 1986-1995.

5. Arnett FC, Edworthy SM, Bloch DA, et al. (1988) The American Rheumatism Association 1987 revised criteria for the classification of rheumatoid arthritis. Arthritis Rheum, 31: 315-324

6. Arosio P, Levi S, Gabri E, et al (1984) Heterogeneity of ferritin II: immunological aspects. In: Albertini A, Arosio P, Chiancone E, Drysdale J (eds) Ferritins and isoferritins as biochemical markers. Elsevier, Amsterdam New York Oxford, 33-47

7. Ascherio A, Rimm EB, Giovanucci E, Willet WC, Stampfer MJ (2001) Blood donation and risk of coronary heart disease. CIRCULATION: 103: 52-57

8. Ascherio A, Willett WC, Rimm EB, Giovanucci E, Stampfer MJ (1994) Diatory iron intake and risk of coronary disease among men. CIRCULATION: 89: 969-974

9. Baker EN, Lindley PF (1992) New perspectives on the structure and function of transferrin. J Inorg Biochem 47: 147-160

10. Baynes RD (1994) Iron Deficiency in Iron Metabolism in Health and Disease (eds. Brock JH, Halliday JW, Pippard MJ, Powell LW) W.B. Saunders Co., 189-198

11. Baynes RD, Skikne BS, Cook JD (1994) Circulating transferrin receptors and assessment of iron status. J Nutr Biochem 5: 322-330.

12. Baynes RD (1996) Assessment of iron status. Clin Biochem 29: 209 – 215

13. Begemann H, Rastetter J (1993) Klinische Hämatologie, 4. Aufl. Thieme, Stuttgart New York

14. Beguin Y (1998) Prediction of response to treatment with recombinant human erythropoietin in anemia associated with cancer. Med Oncol 15 (Suppl. 1): 38-46.

15. Beguin Y (1992) The soluble transferrin receptor: biological aspects and clinical usefulness as quantitative measure of erythropoiesis. Haematologica 77: 1-10

16. Beguin Y et al (1993) Quantitative asessment of erythropoiesis and functional classification of anemia based on measurement of serum transferrin receptor and Erythropoietin. Blood 81: 1067

17. Beguin Y (1992) The soluble transferrin receptor: biological aspects and clinical usefulness as quantitative measure of erythropoiesis. Hematologica 77: 1-10

18. Besarab A, et al. (1998) The effect of normal as compared with low hematocrit values in patients with cardiac disease who are receiving hemodialysis and Erythropoietin. N Engl J Med 339: 584 - 590

19. Beutler E (1997) Genetic irony beyond haemochromatosis: clinical effects of HLA-H mutations. Lancet 349: 296-297

20. Bobbio-Pallavicini F, et al. (1989) Body iron status in critically ill patients: significance of serum ferritin. Int Care Med 15: 171-178

21. Boelaert JR, Weinberg GA, Weinberg ED (1996) Altered iron meta-bolism in HIV infection: Mechanisms, possible consequences and proposals for management. Inf Dis Agents 5: 36-46

22. Bothwell TH, et al. (1989) Nutritional iron requirements and food iron absorption. J Intern Med 226: 357-365

23. Brock JH (1994) Iron in infection, immunity, inflamation and neo-plasia in Iron Metabolism in Health and Disease; ed Brock JH, Halliday JW, Pippard MJ, Powell LW London, W.B. Saunders, pp 353-389

24. Brouwer DAJ, Welten HTME, et al. (1998) Plasma folic acid cutoff value, derived from its relationship with homocyst(e)ine. Clin Chem 44/7: 1545-1550

25. Brugnara C (2000) Reticulocyte Cellular Indices: A New Approach in the Diagnosis of Anemias and Monitoring of Erythropoietic Function. Critical Reviews in Clin Lab Sciences; 37 (2): 93-130

26. Bunn HF (1991) Anemia associated with chronic disorders. In: Harrison's principles of internal medicine, 12th ed., McGraw-Hill, New York, 1529-1531

27. Burns DL, Pomposelli JJ (1999) Toxicity of parenteral iron dextran therapy. Kid Int 55 (Suppl 69): 119-124

28. Carr H, Rodak BF (1999) Clinical hematology atlas. W. B. Saunders, Philadelphia

29. Carmel R (1997) Cobalamin, the stomach and aging. Am J Clin Nutr 66: 750-9

30. Cazzola M, Mercuriali F, Brugnara C, et al. (1997) Use of recombinant human Erythropoietin outside the setting of uraemia. Blood. 89: 4248-4267

31. Cazzola M, et al. (1996) Defective iron supply for erythropoiesis and adequate endogenous Erythropoietin production in anemia associated with systemic onset invenile chronic arthritis. Blood 87: 4824 – 4830

32. Cazzola M, Ponchio L, Pedrotti C, et al. (1996) Prediction to response of recombinant human Erythropoietin (rh-EPO) in anaemia of malignancy. Haematologica. 81: 434-441

33. Cheung W, Minton N, Gunawardena K, et al. (2000) The pharmacokinetics and pharmadynamics of Epoietin Alfa once weekly versus Epoietin Alfa 3 times weekly. Am Soc Haematol; posterpresentation Dec. 4th.

34. Chiancone E, Stefanini F (1984) Heterogeneity of ferritin I structural and functional aspects. In: Albertini A, Arosio P, Chiancone E, Drysdale J (eds) Ferritins and isoferritins as biochemical markers. Elsevier, Amsterdam New York Oxford, pp 23-31

35. Cook JD, et al. (1993) Serum transferrin receptor. Ann Rev Med 44: 63

36. Cook JD, Skikne BS, Baynes RD (1986) Serum transferrin receptor. Blood 687: 726-731

37. Cook JD, Skikne BS (1989) Iron deficiency: Definition and diagnosis. J Intern Med 226: 349-355.

38. Cook JD (1982) Clinical evaluation of iron deficiency. Semin Hematol 19: 6-18.

39. Corti MC, Gaziano M, Hennekeus CH (1997) Iron status and risk of cardiovascular disease. Ann Epidemiol 7: 62-68

40. Covell AM, Worwood M (1984) Isoferritins in plasma. In: Albertini A, Arosio P, Chiancone E, Drysdale J (eds) Ferritins and isoferritins as biochemical markers. Elsevier, Amsterdam New York Oxford, pp 49-65

41. Danielson BG, Salmonson T, Derendorf H, Geisser P (1996) Pharmacokinetics of iron(III)-hydroxide sucrose complex after a single intravenous dose in healthy volunteers. Arzneimittelforschung/Drug Res 46 (I) 6

42. De Jong G, von Dijk IP, van Eijk HG (1990) The biology of transferrin. Clin Chim Acta 190: 1-46

43. De Sousa M, Reimao R, Porto G, et al. (1992) Iron and Lymphocytes: Reciprocal regulatory interactions.
Curr Stud Hematol Blood Transf 58: 171-177

44. Deinhard AS, List A, Lindgren B, Hunt JV, Chang PN (1986) Cognitive deficits in iron-deficient and iron-deficient anaemic children. J Paediatr 108: 681-689

45. Deutsch E, Geyer G, Wenger R (1992) Folsäure-Resorptionstest. In: Laboratoriumsdiagnostik. Wissenschaftliche Buchreihe, Schering, 91-93

46. Dietzfelbinger H (1993) Korpuskuläre hämolytische Anämien. In: Begemann H, Rastetter J (Hrsg) Klinische Hämatologie, 4. Aufl. Thieme, Stuttgart New York, 248-252

47. Dinant JC, de Kock CA, van Wersch JWJ (1995) Diagnostic value of C-reactive protein measurement does not justify replacement of the erythrocyte sedimentation rate in daily general practice. Eur J Clin Invest 25; 353-9

48. Doss M (1998) Porphyrie. In: Thomas L (Hrsg) Labor und Diagnose. TH-Books, Frankfurt/Main 458-470

49. Drysdale JW (1977) Ferritin phenotypes: structure and metabolism. In: Jacobs A (ed) Iron metabolism. Ciba Foundation Symposium 51 (excerpta medica). Elsevier, Amsterdam, pp 41-57

50. Elliot MJ, Maini RN (1994) Repeated therapy with monoclonal antibody to tumor necrosis factor alpha (cA2) in patients with rheumatoid arthritis. Lancet 344: 1125-1127

51. Egrie JC, Dwyer E, Lykos M, et al. (1997) Novel erythropoiesis stimulting protein (NESP) has a longer serum half-life and greater in viro biological activity compared to recombinant human erythropoietin (rHU EPO). Blood 90: 56 A (abstr.)

52. Egrie JC, Grant JR, Gillias DK, Aoki KH, et al. (1993) The Role of Carbohydrate on the Biological Activity of Erythropoietin. Glycoconjugate Journal; 10: S 7.7 (abstr.)

53. Eschbach JW, Haley NR, Adamson JW (1990) The anemia of chronic renal failure: pathophysiology and effects of recombinant Erythropoietin. Contrib Nephrol 78: 24-37

54. Feelders RA, Kuiper-Kramer EPA, van Eijk HG (1999) Structure, function and clinical significance of transferrin receptors. Clin Chem Lab Med 37: 1-10

55. Ferguson BJ, Skikne BS, Simpson KM, Baynes RD, Cook JD (1992)

Serum transferrin receptor distinguishes the anemia of chronic disease from iron deficiency anemia. J Lab Clin Med 19: 385-390

56. Finlayson NDC (1990) Hereditary (primary) hemochromatosis. BMJ 301: 350-351

57. Flowers CH, Skikne BS, Covell AM, Cook JD (1989) The clinical measurement of serum transferrin receptor. J Lab Clin Med 114: 368-377.

58. Folkman J (1997) Addressing tumor blood vessels. Nat Biotechnol; 15: 110-115.

59. Franco RS (1987) Ferritin. In: Pesce AJ, Kaplan LA (eds) Methods in clinical chemistry. CV Mosby Company, St. Louis Washington Toronto, pp 1240-1242

60. Frishman WH (1998) Biologic Markers as Predictors of Cardiovascular Disease. Am J Med; 104: 18s-27s

61. Gabrilove JL, et al. (1999) Once weekly dosing of Epoietin Alfa is similar to three times weekly dosing in increasing Hemoglobin and quality of life. Proc ASCO; Vol. 18: 2216 (abstr)

62. Gargano G, Polignano G, De Lena M, et al. (1999) The utility of a growth factor: rHU-EPO as a treatment for pre-operative autologous blood donation in gynaecological tumor surgery. Int J Oncol; Vol. 4 (1): 157-160.

63. Garry PJ (1984) Ferritin. In: Hicks JM, Parker KM (eds) Selected analytes in clinical chemistry. American Association for Clincal Chemistry Press, Washington, pp 149-153

64. Goldberg MA, Dunning SP, Bunn HF (1988) Regulation of the Erythropoietin gene: evidence, that the oxygen sensor is a hemo protein. Science 24w: 1412-1415

65. Graf H, Lacombe JL, Braun J, et al. (2000) Novel Erythropoiesis stimulating Protein (NESP) for maintains Hemoglobin (Hgb) at a reduced dose frequency compared to recombinant human erythropoietin (EPO) in ESRD patients. Abstr. EDTA 2000

66. Graf H, Lacombe JL, Braun J, Gomes da Costa AA and the European/Australian NESP 980140/194 Study Group (2000) Am Soc Nephr; 33rd Annual Meeting, Toronto (abstr.)

67. Graziadei I, Gaggl S, Kaserbacher R, Braunsteiner H, Vogl W (1994) The acute phase protein alpha-1 antitrypsin inhibits growth and proliferation on human early erythroid progenitor cells and of human erythroleucemic cells by interfering with transferrin iron uptake. Blood 83: 260-268

68. Greendyke RM, Sharma K, Gifford FR (1994) Serum levels of erythro-poietin and selected cytokines in patients with anemia of chronic disease. Am Clin Path 101: 338-341

69. Grützmacher P, Ehmer B, Messinger D, et al. (1991) Therapy with recombinant human Erythropoietin (rEPO) in hemodialysis pati-ents with transfusion dependent anemia. Report of a European mul-ticenter trial. Nephrologia 11: 58-65

70. Gunshin H, Mackenzie B, Berger UV, et al. (1997) Cloning and char-acterization of a mammalian proton-coupled metal-ion transporter. Nature 388: 482 488

71. Hastka J, Lasserre JJ, et al. (1992) Washing erythrocyte to remove interferents in measurements of zinc protoporphyrin by front-face hematofluorometry. Clin Chem 11: 2184-2189

72. Haupt H, Baudner S (1990) Chemie und klinische Bedeutung der Human Plasma Proteine. Behring Institut Mitteilungen 86: 1-66

73. Haverkate F, Thompson SG, et al. (1997) Production of C-reactive protein and risk of coronary events in stable and unstable angina. Lancet 349: 462-466

74. Heidelberger M, Kendall FE (1935) The precipitin reaction between type III pneumococcus polysaccharide and homologous antibody III. A quantitative study and theory of the reaction mechanism. J Exp Med 61: 563-591

75. Heil W, Koberstein R, Zawta B (2000) Referenzbereiche für Kinder und Erwachsene, Präanalytik. Roche Diagnostics GmbH, Mannheim

76. Heinrich HC (1986) Bioverfügbarkeit und therapeutische Wirksam-keit oraler Eisen (^{2})- und (^{3}) Präparate. Schweiz. Apotheker-Zeitung 22: 1231-1256

77. Heinrich HC (1980) Diagnostischer Wert des Serumferritins für die Beurteilung der Gesamtkörper-Eisenreserven. In: Kaltwasser JP, Werner E (Hrsg) Serumferritin. Springer, Berlin Heidelberg New York, S 58-95

78. Henke M, Guttenberger R, Barke A, et al. (1999) Erythropoietin for patients undergoing radiotherapy: a pilot study. Radiother Oncol; Vol 50 (2): 185-190

79. Henry DH, Abels RI (1994) Recombinant human Erythropoietin in the treatment of cancer and chemotherapy-induced anemia: results of double-blind and open label follow-up studies. Semin Oncol 21 [2 Suppl 3]: 21-28

80. Herrmann W, Schorr H, Purschwitz K, Rassoul F, Richter V (2001) Total Homocysteine, Vitamin B12, and Total Antioxidant Status in Vegetarians. Clin Chem 47:6 1094-1101

81. Hermann W, et al. (1997) The Importance of Hyperhomocysteinemia in High Age People. Clin Lab; 43: 1005-1009

82. Hershko CH, Konijin AM (1981) Serum ferritin in hematologic disorders. In: Albertini A, Arosio P, Chiancone E, Drysdale J (eds) Ferritins and isoferritins as biochemical markers. Elsevier, Amsterdam New York Oxford, pp 143-158

83. Hilman RS, Finch CA (1985) Red Cell Manual. 5th Ed., Davis, Philadelphia

84. Hörl WH, Cavill I, et al. (1995) How to get the best out of r-HuEPO? Nephrol Dial Transplant 10 (Suppl 2): 92-95

85. Hörl WH, Cavill I, Macdougall IC, Schaefer RM, Sunder-Plassmann G (1996) How to diagnose and correct iron deficiency during rhEPO therapy, a consensus report. Nephrol Dial Transplant 11: 246-250

86. Hörl WH (2001), Persönliche Mitteilung

87. Huebers HA, Beguin Y, Pootrakne P, Einspahr D, Finch CA (1990) Intact transferrin receptors in human plasma and their relation to erythropoiesis. Blood 75: 102-107

88. International Committee for Standardisation in Haematology (1988) Recommendations for measurement of serum iron in blood. Int J Hematol 6: 107-111

89. Jacobs A, Hodgetts J, Hoy TG (1984) Functional aspects of isoferritins. In: Albertini A, Arosio P, Chiancone E, Drysdale J (eds) Ferritins and isoferritins as biochemical markers. Elsevier, Amsterdam New York Oxford, pp 113-127

90. Jacobs A, Worwood M (1975) Ferritin in serum. N Engl J Med 292: 951-956

91. Jazwinska EC, et al. (1996) Haemochromatosis and HLAH. Nature Genet 14: 249-251

92. Johannsen H, Gross AJ, Jelkmann W (1989) Erythropoietin production in malignancy. In: Jelkmann W, Gross AJ (eds) Erythropoietin. Springer, Berlin Heidelberg New York Tokyo, pp 80-91

93. Johnson AM (1996) Ceruloplasmin. In: Ritchie RF, Navolotskaia O, eds. Serum proteins in clinical medicine. Scarborough: Foundation for Blood Research, 13.01-1-8

94. Jouanolle AM, et al. (1996) Haemochromatosis and HLA-H. Nature Genet 14: 251-252

95. Kaltwasser IP, Werner E (Hrsg) (1980) Serumferritin: Methodische und klinische Aspekte. Springer, Berlin Heidelberg New York

96. Kaltwasser JP, Hörl WH, Cavill J, Thomas L (1999) Anaemia, novel concepts in renal and rheumatoid disease, IFCC-Worldlab-Abstracts, Florence

97. Kaltwasser JP, Werner E (1980) Serumferritin als Kontrollparameter bei der Therapie des Eisenmangels. In: Kaltwasser JP, Werner E (Hrsg) Serumferritin: Methodische und klinische Aspekte. Springer, Berlin Heidelberg New York, S 137-151

98. Kaltwasser JP, Kessler U, Gottschalk R, Stucki G, Möller B (2001) Effect of rHU-Erythropoietin and i.v. Iron on Anaemia and Disease Activity in Rheumatoid Arthritis. J Rheumatol 28: 2430-2437

99. Kessler U, Gottschalk R, Stucki G, Kaltwasser JP (1998) Benefit in clinical outcome and disease activity of treatment of anaemia of chronic diseases in rheumatoid arthritis with recombinant human Erythropoietin. J Rheumatol 41: 210

100. Kiechl S, Willeit J, et al. (1997) Body iron stores and the risk of carotid atherosclerosis: Prospective results from the Bruneck Study. Circulation 96: 3300-3307

101. Knekt P, Revanen A, et al. (1994) Body iron stores and the risk of cancer. Int J Cancer 56: 379-382

102. Köhler G, Milstein C (1975) Continuous cultures of fused cells secreting antibody of predefined specificity. Nature 256: 495

103. Kolbe-Busch S, Lotz J, Hafner G, Blanckaert J, Claeys G, Togni G, Carlsen J, Röddiger R, Thomas L (2002) Multicenter Evaluation of a Fully Mechanized Soluble Transferrin Receptor Assay on the Hitachi and COBAS INTEGRA Analyzers and Determination of Reference Ranges. Clin. Chem. Lab. Med. (acceptet 2002)

104. Krainer M, Fritz E, Kotzmann H, et al. (1990) Erythropoietin modulates lipid metabolism. Blut 61: Abstr No 81

105. Kubota K, Tamura J, et al. (1993) Evaluation of increased serum ferritin levels in patients with hyperthyroidism. Clin.Invest 72 : 26-29

106. Leedma PJ, Stein AR, et al. (1996) Thyroid hormone modulates the interaction between iron regulatory proteins and the ferritin mRNA iron responsive element. J Biol. Chem. 271: 12017-12023

107. Lejeune FJ, Ruegg C, Lienard D (1998) Clinical applications on TNF-alpha in cancer. Curr Opin Immunol 10: 573-580

108. Leon P, Jimence M, Barona P, Sierrasesumaga L (1998) Recombinant human erythropoietin for the treatment of anemia in children with solid malignant tumors. Med Pediatr Oncol; Vol. 30 (2): 110-116

109. Liebelt EI (1998) in: Clinical Management of Poisoning and Drug Overdose. WB Saunders 757-766

110. Lindenbaum J (1988) Neuropsychiatric disorders caused by cobalamin deficiency in the absence of anemia or macrocytosis. N Engl J Med 318: 1720-1728

111. Linke R, Küppers R (1989) Nicht-isotopische Immunoassays - Ein Überblick. In: Borsdorf R, Fresenius W, Günzler H, et al. (Hrsg) Analytiker-Taschenbuch, Bd 8. Springer, Berlin Heidelberg New York Tokyo, S 127-177

112. Linkesch W (1986) Ferritin bei malignen Erkrankungen. Springer, Wien New York

113. Linker CH (2000) Blood in Current Diagnosis and Treatment. 39th Ed.: 505-507

114. Lipschitz DA, Cook JD, Finch CA (1974) A clinical evaluation of serum ferritin as an index of iron stores. N Engl J Med 290: 1213-1218

115. Littlewood TJ, Bajetta E, Nortier JW, Vercammen E, Rapoport B (2001) Epoetin Alfa Study Group: Effects of epoetin alfa on hematologic parameters and quality of life in cancer patients receiving nonplatinum chemotherapy: results of a randomized, double-blind, placebo-controlled trial. J Clin Oncol; 19 (11): 2865-2874

116. Liuzzo G, Biasucci LM, Gallimore JR, et al. (1994) The prognostic value of C-reactive protein and serum amyloid A protein in severe unstable angina. N Engl J Med, 331: 417-424

117. Ludwig H, Chott A, Fritz E (1995) Increase of bone-marrow cellurarity during Erythropoietin treatment in myeloma. Stem Cells (Dayton) 13: [Suppl 2] 77-87

118. Ludwig H, Fritz E, Leitgeb C, Pecherstorfer M, et al. (1994) Prediction of response to Erythropoietin treatment in chronic anemia of cancer. Blood 84: 1056-1063

119. Ludwig H, Leitgeb C, Pecherstorfer M, et al. (1994) Recombinant human Erythropoietin for the correction of anemia in various cancers. Br J Haematol 87 [Suppl 1]: 158 Abstr No 615

120. MacDougall IC, Gray SJ, Elston O, et al. (1999) Pharmacokinetics of novel erythropoiesis stimulating protein compared with erythropoietin alfa in dialysis patients. I Am Soc Nephrol 10: 2392-2395

121. Mac Dougall IC, Roberts DE, Neubert P, et al. (1989) Pharmacokinetics of intravenous, intraperitoneal and subcutanous recombinant erythropoietin in patients on CAPD-A rationale for treatment. Contrib Nephrol 76: 112-121

122. Maini RN, Breedveld FC, Kalden JR, et al. (1998) Therapeutic efficacy of multiple intravenous infusions of anti-tumor necrosis factor monoclonal antibody combined with low-dose weekly methotrexate in rheumatoid arthritis. Arthritis Rheum 41: 1552-1563

123. Mangold C (1998) The causes and prognostic significance of low hemoglobin levels in tumor patients. Strahlenther Onkol; Vol 174 (Suppl. 4): 17-19

124. Mantovani G, Ghiani M, Curreli L, et al. (1999) Assessment of the efficacy of two dosages and schedules of human recombinant erythropoietin in prevention and correction of cis-platin induced anemia in cancer patients. Oncol Rep Vol. 6 (2): 421-426

125. Massey AC (1992) Microcytic anemia. Differential diagnosis and management of iron deficient anemia. Med Clin North Am 76: 549 – 566

126. Mast AE, Blinder MA, et al. (1998) Clinical utility of the soluble transferrin receptor and comparison with serum ferritin in several populations. Clin Chem 44: 45-51

127. Means Jr RT, Krantz SB (1992) Progress in understanding the pathogenesis of anemia of chronic disease. Blood 80: 1639-1647

128. Means RT (1995) Pathogenesis of the anemia of chronic disease: A cytokine mediated anemia. Stem. cells (Dayt) 13: 32-37

129. Means RT, Krantz SB (1992) Progression in understanding the pathogenesis of the anemia of chronic disease. Blood 7: 1639-1647

130. Menacci A, Cenci E, et al. (1997) Iron overload alters T helper cell responses to Candida albicans in mice. J Infect Dis 175: 1467-1476

131. Mercuriali F, Gualtieri G, et al. (1994) Use of recombinant human Erythropoietin to assist autologous blood donation by anemic rheumatiod arthritis patients undergoing major orthopedic surgery. Transfusion 34: 501-506

132. Moldawer LL, Copeland EM (1997) Proinflammatory cytokines, nutritional support, and the cachexia syndrome: interactions and therapeutic options. Cancer 79: 1828-1839

133. Mutane J, Piug-Parellada P, Mitjavila MT (1995) Iron metabolism and oxidative stress during acute and chronic phases of experimental inflammation. Effect of iron dextran and desferoxamine. J Lab Clin Med 126: 435-443

134. Nowrousian MR, et al. (1996) Pathophysiology of cancer-related anemia; in Smyth JF, Boogaerts MA, Ehmer BRM (eds): rhErythropoietin in Cancer Supportive Treatment. New York, Dekker, 1996, pp 13-34

135. Nyman M (1959) Serum haptoglobin methodological and clinical studies. Scand J Clin Lab Invest 11 [Suppl 39]

136. O'Neil-Cutting MA, Crosby WH (1986) The effect of antacids on the absorption of simultaneously ingested iron. JAMA 255: 1468-1470

137. Park JE, Lentner MC, Zimmermann RN, et al. (1999) Fibroblast activation protein, a dual specificity serine protease expressed in reactive human tumor stromal fibroblasts. J Biol Chem 274: 36505-36512

138. Paruta S, Hörl WH (1999) Iron and infection. Kidney International 55 (69), 125-130

139. Peeters HRM, et al. (1996) Effect of recombinant human Erythropoietin on anaemia and disease activity in patients with rheumatoid arthritis and anaemia of chronic disease: a randomised placebo controlled double blind 52 weeks' clinical trial. Am Rheum Dis 55: 739-744

140. Peeters HRM, Jongen-Lavrencic M, Bakker CH (1999) Recombinant human Erythropoetin improves health-related quality of life in patients with rheumatoid arthritis and anaemia of chronic disease; utility measures correlate strongly with disease activity measures. Rheumatol Int 18: 201-206

141. Pepys MB (1996) The acute phase response and C-reactive protein. In: Weatherall DJ, Kuller LH, Tracy RP, Shaten J, Meilahn EN. Relation of C-reactive protein and coronary heart disease in the MRFIT nested case control study. Am J Epidemiol, 144: 537-547

142. Pincus T, et al. (1990) Multicenter study of recombinant human Erythropoietin in correction of anemia in rheumatoid arthritis. Am J Med 89: 161-168

143. Pinggera W (1999) Personal communication

144. Ponka P (1997) Tissue-specific regulation of iron metabolism and

heme synthesis: Distinct control mechanisms in erythroid cells. Blood 89: 1-25

145. Ponka P (1999) Cellular iron metabolism. Kidney International, Vol. 55, Suppl. 69, S2-S11

146. Ponka P, Beaumont C, Richardson R (1998) Function and regulation of transferrin and ferritin. Semin Hematol 35: 35-54.

147. Punnonen K, et al. (1997) Serum transferrin receptor and its ratio to serum ferritin in the diagnosis of iron deficiency. Blood 89/3: 1052-1057

148. Punnonen K, Irjala K, Rajamäki A (1994) Iron deficiency anemia is associated with high concentrations of transferrin receptor in serum. Clin Chem 40: 774-776

149. Qvist N, Boesby S, Wolff B, Hansen CP (1999) Recombinant human erythropoietin and hemoglobin concentrations at operation and during the postoperative period. World J Surg; Vol. 23 (1): 30-35

150. Rauramaa R, Vaisanen S, Mercuri M, et al. (1994) Association of risk factors and body iron status to carotid atherosclerosis in middle aged eastern Finnish men. Eur Heart J 15: 1020-1027

151. Refsum AB, Schreiner BBI (1984) Regulation of iron balance by absorption and excretion. Scand J Gastroenterol 19: 867-874

152. Richardson DR, Ponka P (1997) The molecular mechanisms of the metabolism and transport of iron in normal and neoplastic cells. Biochem Biophys Acta 1331: 1-40

153. Rippmann J, Pfizenmaier K, Mattes R, et al. (2000) Fusion of the tissue factor extracellular domain to a tumour stroma specific single-chain fragment variable antibody results in an antigen-specific coagulation-promoting molecule. Biochem J 349: 1-8

154. Ritchey AK (1987) Iron deficiency in children. Update of an old problem. Postgrad Med 82: 59-63

155. Roberts AG, et al. (1997) Increased frequency of the haemochromatosis Cys 282 Tyr mutation in sporadic prophyria cutanea tarda. Lancet 349: 321-323

156. Robinson SH (1990) Degradation of hemoglobin. In: Williams WJ, Beutler W, Erslev AJ, Lichtman MA (eds) Hematology, 4th edn, McGraw-Hill, New York

157. Rosenberg IH, Alpers DH (1983) Nutrional deficiencies in gastrointestinal disease. In: Sleisenger MH, Fordtran JS (eds) Gastrointestinal disease, 3rd edn, Saunders, New York, pp 1810-1819

158. Roth D, Smith RD, Schulman G, et al. (1994) Effects of recombinant human Erythropoietin on renal function in chronic renal failure predialysis patients. Am J Kidney Dis 24: 777-784

159. Rowland TW, Kelleher JF (1989) Iron deficiency in athletes. Insights from high school swimmers. Am J Dis Child 143: 197-200

160. Ruggeri G, Jacobello C, Albertini A, et al. (1984) Studies of human isoferritins in tissues and body fluids. In: Albertini A, Arosio P, Chiancone E, Drysdale J (eds) Ferritins and isoferritins as biochemical markers. Elsevier, Amsterdam New York Oxford, pp 67-78

161. Sandborn WJ, Hanauer SB (1999) Antitumor necrosis factor therapy for inflammatory bowel disease: a review of agents, pharmacology, clinical results and safety. Inflammatory Bowel Diseases 5 (2), 119-133

162. Sassa S (1990) Synthesis of heme. In: Williams WJ, Beutler E, Erslev AJ, Lichtman MA (eds) Hematology, 4th edn, McGraw-Hill, New York, 332-335

163. Schilling RE, Williams WJ (1995) Vitamin B_{12}-Deficiency: under-diagnosed, overtreated? Hosp Pract 30: 47

164. Schultz BM, Freedman ML (1987) Iron deficiency in the elderly. Baillieres Clin Haematol 1: 291-313

165. Schulze-Osthoff K, Ferrari D, Los M, Wesselborg S, Peter ME (1998) Apoptosis signaling by death receptors. Eur J Biochem 254: 439-459

166. Schurek HJ (1992) Oxygen shunt diffusion in renal cortex and its physiological link to Erythropoietin production. In: Pagel H, Weiss C, Jelkmann W (eds) Pathophysiology and pharmacology of Erythropoietin. Springer, Berlin Heidelberg New York Tokyo, pp 53-55

167. Scigalla P, Ehmer B, Woll EM, et al. (1990) Zur individuellen Ansprechbarkeit terminal niereninsuffizienter Patienten auf die Rh-EPO-Therapie. Nieren-Hochdruckerkrankungen 19: 178-183

168. Scott JM, Weir DG (1980) Drug induced megaloblastic change. Clin Haematol 9: 587-606

169. Sears D (1992) Anemia of chronic disease. Med Clin North Am 76: 567 – 579

170. Sempos CT, Looker AC, Gillum RF, McGee DL, Vuong CV, Johnson CL (2000) Serum ferritin and death from all causes and cardiovascular disease: The NHANES II mortality study. AEP 10: 441-448

171. Shapiro HM (1995) Practical flow cytometry 3rd ed. New York, Wiley-Liss

172. Shinozuka N, Koyama J, Anzai H, et al. (2000) Autologous blood transfusion in patients with hepatocellular carcinoma undergoing hepatectomy. Am J Surg; Vol. 179 (1): 42-45

173. Steinberg D, Parthasarathy S, Carew TE, et al. (1989) Beyond cholesterol: modifications of low-density lipoprotein that increase its atherogenicity. N Engl J Med. 320: 915-924

174. Sullivan JL (1996) Perspectives on the iron and heart disease debate. J Clin Epidermial 49: 1345-1352

175. Sunder-Plassmann G, Hörl WH (1996) Eisen und Erythropoietin. Clin Lab 42: 269-277

176. Sunder-Plassmann G, Hörl WH, eds. (1999) Erythropoietin and iron. Clin. Nephrol 47: 141-157

177. Suominen P, et al. (1997) Evaluation of new immunoenzymometric assay for measuring soluble transferrin receptor to detect iron deficiency in anaemic patients. Clin Chem 43/9: 1641-1646

178. Suominen P, Punnonen K, Rajamäki A, Irjala K (1998) Serum transferrin receptor and transferrin receptor-ferritin index identity healthy subjects with subclinical iron deficits. Blood 92: 2934-2939

179. Sweeney PJ, Nicolae D, Ignacio L, et al. (1988) Effect of subcutaneous recombinant human Erythropoietin in cancer patients receiving radiotherapy: final report of randomized open labeled, phase II trial. Brit J Cancer 77 (11): 1996-2002

180. Thomas AJ, Bunker VW, et al. (1989) Iron status of hospitalized and housebound elderly people. Q J Med 70: 175-184

181. Thomas L (Hrsg.) (1998) Labor und Diagnose, 5. Auflage, TH Books Verlagsgesellschaft, Frankfurt

182. Thomas L, Nowrousian MR, Hörl WH, Möller B, Wick M, et al. (2000) Expert Meeting: Clinical assessment of soluble Transferrin Receptor. Frankfurt

183. Thomas L, Heimpel H, Hörl WH, Kirschbaum A, Maier RF, Pinggera W, Schäfer RM, Weisbach V, Weiss G, Wick M, et al. (2001) Expert Meeting: Stufendiagnostik bei Eisenstoffwechselstörungen. Frankfurt

184. Thomas L, Kaltwasser JP, Kuse R, Pinggera W, Scheuermann EH, Wick M (1997) Konsensus Konferenz: Eisensubstitution bei Dialysepatienten unter Erythropoetintherapie. Frankfurt (unpublished)

185. Thorpe SJ, Walker D, Arosio P, Heath A, Cook JD, Worwood M (1997) International collaborative study to evaluate a recombinant

ferritin preparation as an International Standard. Clin Chem 43: 1582-1587

186. Thorstensen K, Romslo I (1993) The transferrin receptor: its diagnostic value and its potential as therapeutic target. Scand J Clin Lab Invest 53 [Suppl 215]: 113-120

187. van Leeuwen MA, van Rijswijk MH, Sluiter WJ, et al. (1997) Individual relationship between progression of radiological damage and the acute phase response in early rheumatoid arthritis. Towards development of a decision support system. J Rheumatol 24: 20-27

188. Vawenterghem P, Barany P, Mann J, European/Australian NESP 970290 Study Group. Novel Erythropoiesis stimulating Protein (NESP) (1999) Maintains Hemoglobin (Hgb) in ESRD patients when administered once weekly or once every other week. Amer Soc Nephr; 32nd Ann. Meeting A1365

189. Waheed A, Parkkila S, Saarnio J, Fleening RE, et al. (1999) Association of HFE protein with transferrin receptor in crypt enterocytes of human duodenum. Proc. Nat. Acad. Sci. USA 96: 1579-1584

190. Wajant H, Pfizenmaier K (2001) Vom Tumornekrosefaktor zum TRAIL-AMAIZe: Antitumoral wirksame Zytokine der zweiten Generation. Onkologie 24 (suppl. 1): 6-10

191. Walczak H, Miller RE, Ariail K, et al. (1999) Tumoricidal activity of tumor necrosis factor-related apoptosis-indusing ligand in vivo. Nat Med 5: 157-163

192. Ware CF, Santee S, Glass E (1998) Tumor necrosis factor-related ligands and receptors. In: Thomson AW (ed): Cytokine Handbook. San Diego, Academic Press, pp. 549-593

193. Weiss G (1999) Iron and anemia of chronic disease. Kidney international 55 (69) 12-17

194. Weiss G, Fuchs D, Hausen A, Reibnegger G, Werner ER, Werner-Felmayer G, Wachter H (1992) Iron modulates interferon gamma effects in the human myelomonocytic cell line THP-1. Exp Hematol 20: 605-610

195. Weiss G, Houston T, Kastner S, Johrer K, Grunewald K, Brock JH (1997) Regulation of cellular iron metabolism by Erythropoietin: Activation of iron-regulatory protein and upregulation of transferrin receptor expression in erythroid cells. Blood 89: 680

196. Weiss G, Wachter H, Fuchs D (1995) Linkage of cell-mediated immunity to iron metabolism. Immunol Today 16: 495-500

197. Weiss G, Werner-Felmayer G, Werner ER, Grunewald K, Wachter H, Hentze MW (1994) Iron regulates nitric oxide synthase activity by controlling nuclear transcription. J Exp Med 180: 969

198. Weiss TL, Kavinsky CJ, Goldwasser E (1982) Characterization of a monoclonal antibody to human Erythropoietin. Proc Natl Acad Sci USA 79: 5465-5469

199. Wick M, Pinggera W (1994) (personal communication)

200. Williams WJ, Beutler E, Ersler AJ, Lichtman MA (eds) (1990) Hematology, 4th edn. McGraw-Hill, New York

201. Worwood M (1980) Serum ferritin. In: Cook JD (ed) Methods in hematology. Churchill Livingstone, New York, pp 55-89

202. Yanagawa S, Hirade K, Ohnota H (1984) Isolation of human Erythropoietin with monoclonal antibodies. J Biol Chem 259: 2707-2710

203. Yap GS, Stevenson MM (1994) Inhibition of in vitro erythropoiesis by soluble mediators of Plasmodium chalandi AS malaria: lack of a major role of interleukin l, TNF alpha and gamma-Interferon. Infect Immun 62: 357-362

Recommended Reading

- Andrews NC (1999) Disorders of iron metabolism. N Engl J Med 341: 1986-1995.
- Begemann H, Rastetter J (1993) Klinische Hämatologie, 4. Aufl. Thieme, Stuttgart New York
- Beutler E, Lichtman MA, Coller BS, Kipps TH (1995) William's Hematology. 5th ed. McGraw-Hill, New York
- Brostoff J (1997) Taschenatlas der Immunologie: Grundlagen, Labor, Klinik. Thieme, Stuttgart, New York
- Burmester G (1998) Taschenatlas der Immunologie: Grundlagen, Labor, Klinik. Thieme, Stuttgart, New York
- Greiling H, Gressner AM (eds) (1995) Lehrbuch der klinischen Chemie und Pathobiochemie, 3. Aufl. Schattauer, Stuttgart New York
- Heil W, Koberstein R, Zawta B (2002) Referenzbereiche für Kinder und Erwachsene, Pre-Analytical Considerations. Roche Diagnostics GmbH, Mannheim
- Kaltwasser IP, Werner E (Hrsg) (1980) Serumferritin: Methodische und klinische Aspekte. Springer, Berlin Heidelberg New York
- Klein J, Horejsi N (1999) Immunology, 2nd edn. Blackwell Science, Oxford Malden Carlton
- Porstmann B (1993) Retikulozyten – Reifung, Analytik, Klinische Bedeutung. Wachholz, Nürnberg
- Sunder-Plassmann G, Hoerl WH, Guest Editors (1999) Kidney International, Vol 55, Suppl 69
- Themel H, Schick HD (1998) Praktische Differentialdiagnostik in Hämatologie und Onkologie. Thieme, Stuttgart, New York
- Thomas L (Hrsg) (1998) Labor und Diagnose, 5. Aufl. TH Books Verlagsgesellschaft, Frankfurt

Subject Index